Doctors' careers

The training, employment and career movement of doctors is of fundamental concern to all those working in and administrating the National Health Service and private medicine within Britain and around the world.

Doctors' Careers makes available to a wide readership, in one volume, the results of a comprehensive survey of medical choices and career progress of doctors qualifying from British medical schools during a decade, from 1974 to 1983. No other survey of this kind has been carried out over a prolonged period of time. This is a unique record of the aspirations, feelings and experiences of a very large group of doctors, during a time of considerable changes in emigration, training for general practice and the position of women doctors. The book deals with these issues, and also the reasons for choosing and changing careers within medicine, postgraduate qualifications, internal migration of doctors within the UK, aspects of some important individual specialties – medicine, surgery, psychiatry and anaesthetics – and the personal opinions of doctors about their training and the career problems of British medicine. The data have important implications for medical staff planning, and this is taken up in an analysis of the employment status of doctors five years after leaving medical school.

Doctors' Careers will interest doctors, educationalists, health service planners and social scientists in the United Kingdom, and in many other countries where similar problems and experiences are encountered.

James Parkhouse has a broad background for this study, having trained and practised as an anaesthetist, in England, the USA and Canada; been responsible for postgraduate teaching and organising of training, as Professor of Anaesthetics in Winnipeg and Manchester; been directly concerned with medical education in general as Postgraduate Dean in Sheffield, and later in Newcastle; and having been involved in many committees and discussions on medical staff planning. He has lately been Director of the Medical Careers Research Group in Oxford.

Doctors' careers

Aims and experiences of medical graduates

James Parkhouse

ROUTLEDGE

London and New York

First published in 1991
by Routledge
2 Park Square, Milton Park, Abingdon, Oxon, OX14 4RN

Simultaneously published in the USA and Canada
by Routledge
a division of Routledge, Chapman and Hall Inc.
270 Madison Ave, New York NY 10016

Transferred to Digital Printing 2005

Wordprocessed by Amy Boyle Word Processing Services

British Library Cataloguing in Publication Data
Parkhouse, James
Doctors' careers.
1. Great Britain. Doctors
I. Title
610.69520941

Library of Congress Cataloging in Publication Data
Parkhouse, James
Doctors' careers: aims and experiences of medical graduates/James Parkhouse.
p. cm.
Includes bibliographical references.
1. Physicians – Great Britain. 2. Medical colleges – Great Britain–Alumni.
3. Medicine – Vocational guidance – Great Britain.
I. Title.
[DNLM: 1. Career Choice. 2. Career Mobility. 3. Education, Medical.
4. Specialties, Medical. W 21 P246d]
R690.P29 1991
610.69'52'0941 – dc20
DNLM/DLC
for Library of Congress 90-8366
CIP

ISBN 0-415-04649-1

Contents

Figures and tables

FIGURES

TABLES

Introduction and acknowledgements

The origins of the work here reported were in Sheffield in the late 1960s when as Postgraduate Dean I became responsible for studies of medical staffing structure planning following the publication of the report of the Royal Commission on Medical Education in 1968 (the Todd Report). This work had been instigated by Sir Charles Stuart-Harris and was carried out in conjunction with Professor J.F. Knowelden and Dr R.A. Dixon of his Department of Public Health and Preventive Medicine. Dr A.D. Clayden was appointed as research assistant, and publications resulted on the attitudes of trainees to the concept of 'general professional training' (Clayden *et al.* 1971), the allocation of pre-registration posts (Clayden and Parkhouse 1971) and an input/output analysis of progression through the NHS training grades (Clayden and Parkhouse 1972).

In 1970 I moved from Sheffield to Manchester, David Clayden moved to Wales and Cynthia McLaughlin took over as research assistant. As well as stimulating a persistent interest in staffing structure planning (see, for example, Parkhouse and McLaughlin 1975b; Parkhouse 1978) the Sheffield work created the interest of doctors' careers and career choices, originally out of a need for data for staffing level modelling, on which the whole of our subsequent work, as described in this book, was founded. Cynthia's contribution to the design and analysis of our first questionnaires provided a sound basis for all that followed. Also, in Manchester, Janet Black, Mavis Howard and Barbara Hambleton did a great deal of work as members of our developing team on searching out names and addresses, mailing and checking questionnaires, and coding replies. From the Christie Hospital we had unstinted support in computing and statistical analysis from Mike Palmer, Brian Farragher and Neil Bullock. The secretarial burden of typing drafts and preparing tables was ably carried by Pat Coventry, Fiona Dinsdale and Pat Sakalas.

My next move was to Newcastle upon Tyne in 1980, and the

transfer of the project was greatly facilitated by discussions with Ian Russell and Peter Philips of the Health Care Research Unit which, under the directorship of Professor David Newell, gave much support. Barbara Hambleton stayed on for a year in Manchester to complete one phase of the work; Peter Philips continued to give help with data processing and Ian Russell's wife Daphne became a part-time member of our research team working on further surveys and on the analysis of comments from respondents. The mainstay of our period of four years in Newcastle was Malcolm Campbell, who joined us as a full-time research associate and brought a highly intelligent and perceptive mind to the problems of programming and analysis for our increasingly complex and voluminous sets of data. His contribution cannot be over-estimated. My secretary, Irene Macdonald, cheerfully and competently coped with our demands in addition to her routine work.

The project's final move was to Oxford in 1980, when we assumed the title 'Medical Careers Research Group', and I must first acknowledge the help and support of Dame Rosemary Rue and Dr Michael Goldacre in facilitating this move and arranging computer facilities. David Ellin took up, after Malcolm Campbell, the full-time post of research associate and all the problems of data transfer, compatibility with new systems, liaison with new colleagues and further computing development to cope with master-coded data fell on his shoulders. It is a tribute to his work over the last five years that many of the data for this book are available, that the computer files are meticulously updated, and maintained, and that a working relationship which is valued by the Department of Health has been established with their Statistics Division. Don Matthews joined the Oxford team part-time to continue work on the later surveys, and after he left us Penny Rhodes took over and developed a special interest in women doctors which is reflected in that part of this book, as well as in her own publications. Elaine Bland set up the secretarial side of things in Oxford, after which Mavis Lowe joined us and became an important member of our team. It is to Mavis that I am especially grateful for so much cheerful and superbly capable work on the typing of drafts, the preparation of difficult tables and the assembly of material for this book.

The person not so far mentioned is my wife, who has been part of the project from the start and who has followed it throughout its evolution. It must always be a special joy to work as a husband and wife team, to share the excitements, the frustrations and burdens of a continuing piece of work. To me it has certainly been a great joy; Hilda, who has probably mailed, checked and coded more questionnaires than anybody else, and who has done much writing of papers and chapters, has also, I know, enjoyed working in all our venues. No thanks of mine for her support could be adequate.

We have had much reason to appreciate the kindness and help of the Department of Health; Mike Abrams, Doreen Rothman and many others have stood by us when this help was needed, and our meetings and discussions over the years have always been valuable and amicable.

I should also like to acknowledge the help of many other organizations: individual medical schools and Royal Colleges, the Examining Boards of the Non-University Qualifying Examinations in England and Scotland, and especially the General Medical Council, who have assisted us on many occasions by responding to our requests for names and addresses and other information.

I write as 'we' in this book, since I act as spokesman for so many people whose friendship and huge amount of work it is impossible for me to acknowledge adequately. The opinions that show through are my own.

Much of the material in some chapters of this book is based on previously published articles: in the *British Medical Journal* (Chapters 3, 8 and 15), *Medical Education* (Chapters 2, 5 and 13), the *Journal of Public Health Medicine*, formerly entitled *Community Medicine* (Chapters 6, 9 and 15), *Health Bulletin* (Chapter 14) and *Update* (Chapter 14). I am grateful to the editors of these journals for permission to use this material, and to Professor J.K. Galbraith for permission to quote his words on p. 313.

1 The background

The fact that this work on career choices began as a by-product of an interest in medical staffing structure planning gives a fair picture of the relationship between the two pursuits. This introduction sketches some of the relevant things that happened in British medicine during the years before our studies began in the early 1970s, and some of the significant changes that accompanied their continuation into the later 1980s.

Staffing structure planning in medicine has an appeal which was obvious in the UK since the beginning of the National Health Service (NHS) (Parkhouse 1978) and has become an attractive idea to other countries more recently. In theory, one can train the right number of doctors, distribute them appropriately and thus provide a good standard of medical care without unemployment or waste of money. In practice, this works only up to a point, that point depending on the way the planning is done and the degree to which it can be implemented, which has a lot to do with the way doctors earn their living. Forecasting of supply and demand is one thing; bringing about change is another. With increasing medical specialization — itself a matter of serious interest in many countries (World Health Organization 1985; Parkhouse 1989b) — planning involves not only regulating the total number of medical school places, with or without immigration controls, but also sorting out the kinds of work different numbers of doctors do: by chance, choice, direction of labour or a mixture of all three.

Early efforts at medical staffing level planning after the Second World War assumed that doctors, once trained, would work full-time and pretty hard; some would go abroad to the colonial medical service and elsewhere, and little mention was made of foreign doctors coming in, except from Ireland. By the end of the 1970s the changes in social attitudes and in the relevant assumptions were spectacular. It is no surprise that by the mid-1970s the Department of Health (DoH) was commissioning studies on three major areas of concern: factors determining career choice (Hutt *et al.* 1979), overseas doctors in the NHS (D.J. Smith 1980) and women doctors (Ward 1982).

The consequence of allowing too many doctors to train is potential unemployment, with the related consequences of over-specialization, misuse of skills including excessive treatment, and the brain drain. In the mid-1950s there were already worries that not enough jobs would be available in general practice, and this led indirectly to the Willink Committee's (Willink Report 1957) recommendation that medical school places should be cut by 10 per cent. In the 1980s there have again been fears of medical unemployment, but well-reasoned reports (DHSS 1985; DoH 1989) have seen no good grounds for cutting back a medical school intake which is far above the Willink level. The consequence of not training enough doctors is to create a potential vacuum, abhorred by those in need of medical help. This is exactly what happened after Willink, and what would have happened without it because 10 per cent either way was nothing compared to what the appetite of the NHS for doctors was unobtrusively consuming. Into the vacuum overseas doctors came by the thousand, for postgraduate training or, more realistically, to keep the NHS alive. During the late 1960s and most of the 1970s the number of overseas doctors entering the UK each year, and finding work in the NHS, was much larger than the number qualifying each year from our own medical schools, giving us a net annual gain in the order of 1,500 doctors. So much for general staffing forecasting; a look inside the system revealed bigger problems still. Most overseas doctors — nearly all in fact — occupied junior hospital posts. The numbers of these posts increased out of all proportion to training needs; more and more patient care was given by senior house officers (SHOs) and registrars, up to 50 per cent or more of whom were from abroad. The career structure, which had always been a problem (Parkhouse 1965), was heading for chaos.

While doctor immigration was for some time a rather unnoticed problem, the emigration of British doctors caused much concern. Estimates published in 1961 and 1962 (Davison 1962; Seale 1966) seemed alarmingly high and created controversy. It took meticulous and wide-ranging research, (Abel-Smith and Gales 1964; Gish 1970) to separate fact from fiction, but the conclusion was that Britain was losing, each year, not far short of 1,000 home-produced doctors. Not all of these doctors stayed abroad permanently, of course, any more than all the immigrant doctors remained permanently in Britain; but the permanent loss was equivalent to about a quarter of the whole output of our medical schools. There was no lack of good prospects in a number of welcoming countries for high-quality clinical practice and well-funded research, which to many British doctors offered an attractive alternative to the time-serving stuffiness of the hospital specialties and the often rather self-righteous cheese-paring of academic life at home.

General practice had begun to gain strength after serious confrontations with government in 1965 over terms and conditions of service (Forsyth 1966: ch. 3) resulting in the 'GPs' charter', which offered better financial rewards and much more chance of well-organized and adequately supported practice, increasingly on a small-group basis. The first academic departments with professorships were up and running by the beginning of the 1970s, and although three years of postgraduate training for general practice did not become mandatory in the NHS until the end of that decade, more and more training schemes were developing and being taken up voluntarily during the preceding years. It was not that young doctors had previously gone straight from medical school into general practice; the great majority had always, since the NHS began, looked for some hospital experience first: but whereas the move into general practice had very often resulted from failure to make progress in a preferred hospital career, it came more commonly to be a planned move for positive reasons. This improved status of general practice, which has undoubtedly been coupled with higher standards, was reflected in its rising popularity as a career choice, already evident when our studies began in 1971 and sustained ever since.

The Royal Commission on Medical Education (Todd Report 1968) published its conclusions in 1968, but had already, by way of an interim report, given impetus to a massive reversal of the Willink view — an increase in medical school places from under 2,000 in 1968 to over 4,000 twenty years later. The Todd Report made many other important recommendations which reverberated through the 1970s, particularly regarding postgraduate training. This was a period of optimism and expansion; all of higher education was buoyantly responding to the Robbins Report's (1963) call for more places and new universities; in the medical schools there was a surge of new posts, new departments and newly designated university hospitals. The NHS was prosperous, by more recent standards, and there was hope of better career planning and progress. A series of meetings between government and the medical profession led to 'progress reports' (Report 1969) which laid down a formula for correcting the imbalance between junior and senior hospital posts by allowing only 2.5 per cent growth a year in the junior grades while the consultant grade would expand by 4 per cent a year. All would have been well by 1978 except for the fact that, by then, the junior grades had actually continued to expand far more rapidly than the consultant grade! So much for implementation. Meanwhile, a DHSS programme for redistributing junior posts from well-provided to relatively deprived regions had been abandoned as a total failure because no consultant was willing to surrender a junior post and no power on earth was prepared to try and make him or her do so. Only in 1986, after several years of painful negotiation, was this redistribution exercise revived — tentatively, partially and very slowly — through the Joint Planning Advisory Committee, which also had to deal with the balance between clinical and academic posts in the training grades.

Obviously all was not well with hospital careers. For junior doctors matters reached a crisis amounting to strike proportions in 1976, as a result of which extra duty payments were introduced. This differential system of payment highlighted several dilemmas which continue to niggle within the system: extra money for working too many hours is a poor substitute for having adequate payment for a reasonable working week; in some specialties, such as surgery, junior doctors often want many hours of work at night and at weekends to gain experience, but they should be supervised and taught, and patients should not suffer from their over-enthusiasm and consequent exhaustion; the specialties which attract the fewest extra duty payments are often the ones most lacking in recruits even without the disincentive of lower remuneration; if reducing excessive hours of work is seen as a priority then the 'new' financial arrangements seem inappropriate; and — most important of all — if junior doctors are to work fewer hours then either there must be more of them, which is death to any hope of a decent career structure, or trained specialists must take on more out-of-hours commitments. This last proposition, which is the obvious and only long-term solution, had already been given a chilly reception when put forward by Sir George Godber's Working Party (DHSS 1969).

The mid-1970s saw the beginning of changes in international movement of doctors which have been complex and important. Recognition for registration was withdrawn by the General Medical Council from many medical schools in the Indian subcontinent between 1972 and 1975, and tests of language and medical competence were introduced for overseas doctors in 1975. Opportunities for British doctors abroad were diminishing, as many of the popular countries, such as the USA, Canada, and Australia, began to close their doors or introduce formidable entry tests in response to fears of their own medical unemployment and tightening of their research budgets. Increasing rigidity of postgraduate training requirements deterred many British doctors from stepping aside from the career ladder to work abroad. Entry into the European Community (EC) had little effect and has, in fact, only very recently produced any appreciable rise in movement to and from other countries in the EC. But from the mid-1970s onwards the world has been a smaller place for British medical graduates, while their numbers have grown very greatly. With this and the various changes that have affected overseas doctors intending to enter or remain in the UK, the balance in the junior hospital grades has shifted towards a filling-up of the still too-many posts with home graduates, seeking and reasonably expecting promotion.

The increasing output of British medical schools brought with it a large rise in the number of young women doctors, in proportions amounting to 50 per cent or more of many graduating classes. The fact that these young women, many of whom would naturally bear children, not only would wish to pursue their careers but also would be depended on to do so created concern about equal opportunities which mirrored the general spirit of the times. It forced attention on part-time medical employment. In fact, many doctors had always worked on a casual or part-time basis in the NHS, for instance as locums, clinical assistants and salaried partners in general practice. Although these relatively lowly forms of employment came to be resented by some strongly career-motivated women, their abolition would have been even more strongly resented by many other women, and by men. In any case it is doubtful if the NHS could survive without them. But the point was well made that women doctors should have the *choice*, equally with men, of whether to compete for a consultant or general practice principal appointment or opt for a less demanding grade. How to ensure this choice is a difficult matter in a traditionally competitive profession: at what point does the convenience of a part-time post become a necessity, and at what point does equal opportunity become reverse discrimination? Despite these problems, considerable progress has been made, perhaps especially in regard to part-time postgraduate training — much more than in many other countries or professions. Although shifts in attitudes and practice have certainly not been as great as the more determined activists would wish, the influence of this movement, and its more muted counterpart among men, has been more far-reaching than is often recognized. The view that the medical system needs to be infinitely adaptable to the requirements of the individuals within it, rather than the individuals having to fit in as best they can with the system, may provoke snorts of disgust from reactionaries who like to recall the hardships of their own early days, but time will surely tell.

In 1981 the House of Commons Select Committee (Social Services Committee 1981) produced a report which brilliantly described and illustrated the problems of the career structure, and made good, strong recommendations for improving postgraduate training and patient care. These recommendations, for once, were warmly welcomed by the government, and also by junior doctors; the senior members of the profession, and its influential bodies, were cool, suspicious or frankly critical. Not much actually happened, as the Select Committee itself noted with some acerbity four years later (Social Services Committee 1985). The medical profession's own response to the rising sense that something must be done was embodied in the papers *Achieving a Balance* (DHSS 1986) and *Plan for Action* (DHSS 1987b) — a much more cautious and diplomatic attempt to improve career prospects for British medical graduates without antagonizing the consultant body, by separating a reduced number of 'career' registrar posts from a potentially unlimited number of non-progressing registrar posts if sufficient overseas doctors with good credentials could be found to fill them. As always, the scheme depended first and foremost on substantial consultant expansion, and after a couple of years this had again failed to materialize. By that time the government had diverted attention by disclosing its own views on the future of the NHS as a whole (Secretaries of State for Health 1989). The title *Working for Patients* was viewed sardonically by many as a thin veil over a set of proposals which were mostly concerned with political ideology. Some important positive ideas were there: audit, clinical budgeting, financial reward for efficient hospital care, and improved information services. But these needs were already recognized and the means of implementation were vague. Teaching and research seemed likely to fare badly if the plans were fully pushed through, and thoughts of improved personnel planning and a better career structure were rather at variance with a governmental enthusiasm for 'demand-driven' higher education, and individual hospitals with freedom to make their own terms with doctors at different grades. It seemed that the medical profession's almost infinite capacity for sitting on committees might face a stern test.

To secure the morale and well-being of the NHS not only must the doctors, the nurses and others who work in it believe in it, but also the government must believe in it, with a conviction that rings true. When conviction appears to waver, some will say of the NHS, as of medical staffing structure planning, that we might be better off without it; but others will defend the one, or the other, or both, to their last gasp.

2 The study

The Royal Commission on Medical Education (1968) made quite detailed proposals for General Professional Training — a period of three years following the pre-registration year, during which doctors would gain experience in a variety of specialties, by means of six-month appointments. This would give an opportunity to sample different kinds of medical work and would, for most people, constitute a broad beginning to specialist training, either in hospital or general practice, by providing relevant experience. A number of general professional training packages were suggested, as examples which would be suitable for doctors with various career intentions. It was obviously meant that existing SHO and registrar posts would provide the material for this scheme; the idea of using these posts in a planned and systematic way, and linking them across specialty boundaries, was new.

The Nuffield Provincial Hospitals Trust gave support for a feasibility study, in Sheffield, to see whether the existing numbers and types of junior hospital posts would make the introduction of the general professional training scheme practicable. To model this, it was necessary to know how medical graduates in the years following 1968 were likely to want to distribute themselves among the broad divisions of medical work — the nine 'mainstreams' of the Royal Commission Report: medicine (including the medical specialties and paediatrics), surgery (including the surgical specialties), obstetrics and gynaecology, anaesthetics, psychiatry, pathology, radiology and radiotherapy, general practice, and community medicine. Information was available from an Appendix to the Royal Commission report about the probable career intentions of final-year medical students in 1966, but it was felt that more recent data, and from doctors who had actually qualified, would be useful. Hence our initial interest in career choices.

As an exercise in staffing planning this approach is, educationally speaking, 'demand-driven'; it assumes that the numbers of available jobs of various kinds should be determined by the demands of those seeking them. But caution is needed about the use of words, as well as about the soundness of the approach. In the usual analysis of the supply and demand equation of medical staff, as for example in the reports of the Advisory Committee on Medical Manpower Planning (DHSS 1985; DoH 1989), the 'supply' is the availability of medical graduates entering the profession and the 'demand' is the requirement for doctors to meet the needs of the service and the public. In this sense our feasibility study on general professional training was 'supply' driven; but the much more important question that remains is whether meeting the career aspirations of newly qualified doctors will also, conveniently, meet the specialty needs of the service. This issue comes up repeatedly in later chapters.

In 1971-3 we had ready access to names and addresses of qualifiers from the Sheffield and Manchester medical schools. We surveyed the career choices of the 1971 qualifiers, with an 88.5 per cent response rate (McLaughlin and Parkhouse 1972) and this gave data for computer modelling. There was enough interest in the career choice findings themselves for us to repeat the Sheffield and Manchester survey for 1972 (McLaughlin and Parkhouse 1974) and again for 1973 (Parkhouse and McLaughlin 1975a) qualifiers. We followed up the 1971 qualifiers in 1974 (Parkhouse 1976b), and the 1972 and 1973 qualifiers in 1976 (Parkhouse and Howard 1978), to see what had happened to them and their career intentions. The full details of these early studies have been published. Their main value was to give an indication from two provincial schools of what the general situation might be, and to encourage us, through the high response rates and interest in the results, to launch out on more comprehensive studies. The Sheffield/Manchester surveys already showed the rising popularity of general practice as a first career choice. They also showed that the majority of doctors at the pre-registration stage had not made definite choices, and that many doctors changed their choices during the subsequent three or four years, with a further shift towards general practice. The commonest reasons for change of choice were domestic circumstances, reappraisal of aptitudes and abilities, experience of the new choice of career, and additional knowledge of promotion prospects and difficulties.

In 1975 we sent a questionnaire to qualifiers from all the medical schools in England, Scotland and Wales in the calendar year 1974, asking about career choices. The response rate was 86.1 per cent. The following year we repeated the survey for

Table 2.1 Numbers of questionnaires sent and (uncorrected percentage response rates)

Year of qualifying	Years after qualifying[a] 1		3		5		7		9		11		13	
1974	2,348	(86.1)	1,936	(76.9)	2,314	(76.1)	2,330	(83.6)	2,337	(83.4)	2,324	(79.4)	2,323	(79.2)
1975	2,734	(81.1)	2,146	(79.9)										
1976	2,980	(85.1)	2,472	(81.2)										
1977	3,177	(83.9)	3,170	(74.4)	3,061	(84.0)	3,143	(78.2)	3,136	(81.4)				
1978	3,137	(87.6)												
1979	3,190	(87.1)												
1980	3,419	(83.5)	3,433	(82.1)	3,418	(79.6)								
1983	3,845	(82.1)	3,841	(78.7)										

Note: a Response rates may differ from those shown in earlier publications, because corrections were sometimes made in previous reports for doctors written to but found to be deceased, untraceable or not willing to participate

1975 qualifiers, including Queen's University, Belfast. In 1977 we surveyed the career choices of 1976 qualifiers, and also wrote again to 1974 qualifiers to follow their progress. This pattern of surveying each new year of qualifiers and following up previous cohorts at two-yearly intervals continued until 1979. The new medical schools of Nottingham and Southampton were included as their graduates appeared in 1975 and 1977. By 1979 so much data had accumulated that a decision was taken jointly with the DHSS that after 1980 no further new qualifiers would be surveyed until 1983, and two-yearly follow-up questionnaires would be sent only to each third cohort of qualifiers: those of 1974, 1977, 1980 and 1983. In 1980 the Leicester medical school produced its first qualifiers. Up to 1976 fewer than ten students a year entered the clinical part of the undergraduate course in Cambridge; from 1978 onwards the newly developed Cambridge clinical medical school contributed increasing numbers of qualifiers. Our final questionnaires were sent out in 1986 to 1977 qualifiers and in 1987 to 1974 qualifiers. Table 2.1 gives details of the size and dates of the surveys, with response rates.

Our general policy has always been to keep questionnaires as simple as possible, asking for factual information or relatively simple evaluations of such things as intention of remaining in the UK or the importance of one or more of a list of reasons for career choice or change of choice. There has always been space for individual comment and this has often come in profusion. Additional questions were added to some questionnaires, to obtain information about movement during training, reasons for going abroad and returning, and views on the quality of various aspects of training and its impact on competence. This last topic occasioned the sending of a separate questionnaire to 1974 qualifiers in 1984 — a much more searching and detailed inquiry than usual which produced a lower but still perhaps surprising good response rate of 63.7 per cent (Parkhouse *et al.* 1988). A sample questionnaire is reproduced in the Appendix.

Because of the interest that respondents showed in our surveys we arranged to meet some of them face to face. This was done by way of two two-day meetings at the NHS Training and Studies Centre in Harrogate, the White Hart. The first meeting was in February 1984, and consisted of a group of 1974 qualifiers, who included a lecturer in neurology, a specialist in infectious diseases, a GP ex-trainee in psychiatry, a lecturer in surgery, a senior registrar in paediatrics, a senior registrar in medicine, a senior registrar in anaesthetics, a freelance medical adviser and three principals in general practice. The group who assembled for the second meeting in March 1985 included five of those who had come the year before and six attending for the first time. Spouses (including two doctors) and children were also invited, and the discussions were reinforced by the presence of Professor Arthur Crisp, then Chairman of the Education Committee of the General Medical Council, Dr J.M. Cundy from the BMA, and Drs Doreen Rothman, Christine Swinson and Peter Simpson from the DHSS. Much support was given by Tony Turrill, who, as Principal of the White Hart, made the necessary arrangements, and by Tony Milne, who as a professional counsellor not only expounded his subject but also gave greatly appreciated personal service to many of the participants.

My wife and I also had the great pleasure of meeting very many of the Glasgow University medical graduates of 1974 at their annual reunion in 1984. We were, sadly, unable to accept an equally generous invitation to attend the 1974 Birmingham medical graduates reunion in 1984.

When we began large-scale surveys in 1975 we had no particular long-term aim in mind. Our purpose was to gather up-to-date information about career choices which might be useful. The progression to following-up respondents seemed obvious, if it could be done, in view of the early uncertainties of choice and the potential influence of many factors after leaving medical school. Having found that it could be done, many topical issues came into play such as emigration, women doctors' careers, progress in different specialties, and the employment position of young doctors. All of this has clear implications for personnel planning, but there has been no grand strategy of asking questions for specific purposes in relation to large policy decisions. The primary objective has been to assemble comprehensive data which are good enough in themselves to be applied, or built upon, as circumstances suggest.

DEFINING THE POPULATION

Who are the doctors who qualify to practise medicine in a given year? The first decision to be made is whether to work on the academic year, the calendar year, or the year used by the NHS for its census data on medical staffing, which ends on 30 September. All have disadvantages. We have used the calendar year for our studies.

A further problem is that there are two methods in the UK of qualifying to practise medicine: a university degree or a non-university licensing examination of which there are three: MRCS LRCP (Conjoint), LMSSA (the Society of Apothecaries) and the

Scottish triple qualification. The number of *graduates* is not therefore the same as the number of *qualifiers*. Some students take both university and non-university examinations, so that double counting is possible. The two examinations may not be taken in the same calendar year, or academic year; thus, among people who graduate MB ChB in a given year, some may already have become qualified to practise medicine in a previous year. Again, a university degree may not actually be awarded until the year after the year in which the course was completed and the examinations were taken.

Information obtained from individual medical schools may be confusing because students sometimes transfer from one school to another, or they may fall back for health reasons, or to re-sit examinations, or take an intercalated year to obtain an additional degree in a science related to medicine. Oxford and Cambridge medical graduates had very often, particularly before the development of the clinical school in Cambridge, been clinical students elsewhere, most often at one of the London teaching hospitals. University pass lists show only graduates. Lists of qualifiers are obtainable from the non-university licensing bodies, but they do not show who also has a university qualification and do not always give the medical school from which candidates have entered. Many entrants to these examinations are from overseas medical schools; our studies were concerned only with doctors whose undergraduate training was in the UK, but there is yet another small problem about students from abroad who for political reasons complete their undergraduate course in the UK. This occurred with some Maltese students among our 1974 qualifiers.

Another means of identifying qualifiers is to scan the General Medical Council's lists of doctors obtaining provisional registration in order to start the pre-registration year. These lists are produced every two weeks; they give the medical school and the actual date of qualification. The obvious limitation is that doctors who do not choose to register with the GMC are missed.

We made an analysis of this complex situation for two of our cohorts — the qualifiers of 1977 and 1983 (Parkhouse and Parkhouse 1989b) since, during this period, some changes had occurred. The analysis is shown in Tables 2.2 to 2.5 and the main conclusions are summarized below.

Table 2.2 Non-London medical schools (1977 qualifiers)

Clinical medical school	*Same univ.*	*University graduates from clinical school*			*Non-univ. qualifn only*	*Drs with previous qualifn*	*First-time qualifiers*	*MCRG list 1986*	*Drs not on MCRG list*[a]			*No. of grads on univ. list*
		Oxfd	*Camb.*	*Lond.*					*GMC reg.*	*Not GMC Reg. ? UK*	*? foreign*	
Aberdeen	101	–	–	–	–	–	101	101	–	–	–	101
Dundee	100	–	–	–	–	–	100	100	–	–	–	100
Edinburgh	148	–	–	–	–	–	148	147	–	1	–	148
Glasgow	280	–	–	–	2	–	282	281	1[b]	–	–	280
Birmingham	153	–	–	–	1	–	154	153	–	–	1	153
Bristol	125	–	–	1	3	1	128	127	–	1	–	125
Leeds	107	–	–	–	–	–	107	106	1[c]	–	–	107
Liverpool	125	–	–	1	6	1	131	131	–	–	–	125
Manchester	220	–	–	–	2	–	222	219	1[d]	–	2	220
Newcastle	107	–	2	–	1	–	110	110	–	–	–	107
Nottingham	42	–	–	–	–	–	42	42	–	–	–	42
Sheffield	110	–	–	–	1	–	111	110	1[e]	–	–	110
Southampton	64	–	–	–	–	–	64	63	–	–	1	64
Cambridge	–	–	3	–	3	2	4	4	–	–	–	167[f]
Oxford	–	62	–	–	–	–	62	61	1[g]	–	–	79

Table 2.2 continued

Clinical medical school	*Same univ.*	*University graduates from clinical school*			*Non-univ. qualifn only*	*Drs with previous qualifn*	*First-time qualifiers*	*MCRG list 1986*	*Drs not on MCRG list*[a]			*No. of grads on univ. list*
		Oxfd	*Camb.*	*Lond.*					*GMC reg.*	*Not GMC Reg. ? UK*	*Not GMC Reg. ? foreign*	
Wales	125	–	1	–	2	–	128	128	–	–	–	126[h]
Belfast	139	–	–	–	–	–	139	138	1	–	–	139
Total c/f	1,946	62	6	2	21	4	2,033	2,021	6	2	4	2,192[i]

Notes: a Not including doctors with previous qualifications
b No prov. reg. Full reg. Dec 1980
c Prov. reg. 1979
d Prov. reg. July 1977
e Prov. reg. July 1977
f Includes one with Wales degree also
g Prov. reg. Jan. 1977
h Includes one with Cambridge degree also
i Corrected for double count of graduate with Cambridge and Wales degrees

Source: Parkhouse and Parkhouse 1989b

Table 2.3 London medical schools and totals (1977 qualifiers)

Clinical medical school	University graduates from clinical school			Non-univ. qualifn only	Drs with previous qualifn	First-time qualifiers	MCRG list 1986	Drs not on MCRG list[a]			No. of grads on univ. list
								GMC reg.	Not GMC Reg.		
	Oxfd	Camb.	Lond.						? UK	? foreign	
Charing Cross	–	6	47	4	2	55	55	–	–	–	47
Guy's	1	13	100	12	10	116	116	–	–	–	100
King's College	3	38	64	5	–	110	109	–	–	1	64
The London	–	17	80	–	1	96	96	–	–	–	80
Middlesex	1	17	102	1	–	121	119	2[b]	–	–	102
Royal Free	–	–	81	12	2	91	91	–	–	–	81
St Bart's	–	6	113	8	4	123	122	1[c]	–	–	113
St George's	–	17	34	2	–	53	53	–	–	–	34
St Mary's	–	6	82	9	5	92	91	–	1	–	82
St Thomas'	11	18	65	3	6	91	91+1[d]	–	–	–	65
UCH	1	3	104	4	2	110	109	–	1	–	104
Westminster	–	18	46	4	2	66	65	–	1	–	46
London total	17	159	918	64	34	1,124	1,117	3	3	1	920[e]
Total b/f	62	6	2	21	4	2,033	2,021	6	2	4	2,192

Table 2.3 continued

Clinical medical school	*University graduates from clinical school*			*Non-univ. qualifn only*	*Drs with previous qualifn*	*First-time qualifiers*	*MCRG list 1986*	*Drs not on MCRG list*[a]			*No. of grads on univ. list*
	Oxfd	*Camb.*	*Lond.*					*GMC reg.*	*Not GMC Reg. ? UK*	*? foreign*	
Unknown	–	2	–	–	–	2	–	–	2	–	–
Total	79	167	920	85	38	3,159	3,138[f]	9	7	5	3,112

3,112 University graduates
+85 Non-university qualifiers

3,197
-38 Doctors with previous qualifications

3,159 Doctors qualifying for the first time in 1977
-21 Doctors not listed by MCRG

3,138 Doctors on MCRG list plus one who graduated in 1976

Notes: a Not including doctors with previous qualifications
c Prov. reg. Jan. 1977
e Includes two students at English provincial medical schools
b One with no prov. reg. Full reg. 1979. One with prov. reg. May 1977
d List includes one 1976 graduate
f Plus one 1976 graduate

Source: Parkhouse and Parkhouse 1989b

Table 2.4 Non-London medical schools (1983 qualifiers)

Clinical medical school	*University graduates same univ.*	*University graduates other univ.*	*Non-univ. qualifn only*	*Drs with previous qualifn*	*First-time qualifiers*	*MCRG list 1986*	*Drs not on MCRG list*[a] *GMC reg.*	*Drs not on MCRG list*[a] *Not GMC reg. ? UK*	*Drs not on MCRG list*[a] *Not GMC reg. ? foreign*	*No. of grads on univ. list*
Aberdeen	110	–	–	–	110	110	–	–	–	110
Dundee	104	–	–	–	104	104	–	–	–	104
Edinburgh	146	–	–	–	146	141	1[b]	–	4	146
Glasgow	183	–	–	–	183	183	–	–	–	183
Birmingham	152	–	–	–	152	152	–	–	–	152
Bristol	128	–	2	–	130	129	–	1	–	128
Leeds	151	1[c]	–	–	152	152	–	–	–	151
Leicester	99	–	–	–	99	99	–	–	–	99
Liverpool	125	–	1	–	126	126	–	–	–	125
Manchester	228	–	2	–	230	230	–	–	–	228
Newcastle	133	–	–	–	133	133	–	–	–	133
Nottingham	109	–	–	–	109	109	–	–	–	109
Sheffield	139	–	3	–	142	142	–	–	–	139
Southampton	119	–	1	–	120	120	–	–	–	119
Cambridge	81	5[d]	2	5	83	81	2[e]	–	–	128
Oxford	86	–	1	–	87	87	–	–	–	86

Table 2.4 continued

Clinical medical school	University graduates same univ.	other univ.	Non-univ. qualifn only	Drs with previous qualifn	First-time qualifiers	MCRG list 1986	Drs not on MCRG list[a] GMC reg.	Not GMC reg. ? UK	? foreign	No. of grads on univ. list
Wales	133	–	1	–	134	134	–	–	–	133
Belfast	171	–	–	–	171	171	–	–	–	171
Total c/f	2,397	6	13	5	2,411	2,403	3	1	4	2,444

Notes: a Not including doctors with previous qualifications
c Cambridge degree and LMSSA (1983)
e Provisional registration only
b Not in 1984 Medical Register
d Previous qualifiers – medical school not identified

Source: Parkhouse and Parkhouse 1989b

Table 2.5 London medical schools and totals (1983 qualifiers)

Clinical medical school	1983 University graduates London	Camb.	Other	Non-univ. qualifn only	Drs with previous qualifn	First-time qualifiers 1983 only	Incl. Jan 1984	MCRG list 1986	Drs not on MCRG list[a] GMC reg.	Not GMC reg. ? UK	? foreign	No. of grads on 1983 univ. list
Charing Cross	119	–	–	2	–	121	138	137	1[b]	–	–	119
Guy's/St Thomas'	214	18	–	12	12	232	240	240	–	–	–	214
King's	110	2	–	–	6	106	117	116	1[c]	–	–	110
The London	103	6	–	3	1	111	126	126	–	–	–	103
Middlesex	113	6	–	1	–	120	127	127	–	–	–	113
Royal Free	101	–	–	3	1	103	105	105	–	–	–	101
St Bart's	144	3	–	6	1	152	167	167	–	–	–	144
St George's	90	2	–	–	–	92	96	96	–	–	–	90
St Mary's	104	–	–	–	1	103	116	116	–	–	–	104
UCH	101	1	–	–	–	102	115	115	–	–	–	101
Westminster	86	3	–	1	–	90	96	96	–	–	–	86
London total	1,285	41	–	28	22	1,332	1,443	1,441	2	–	–	1,285
Total b/f	–	6	2,397	13	5	2,411	2,411	2,403	3	1	4	2,444
Total	1,285	47	2,397	41	27	3,743	3,854	3,844	5	1	4	3,729

Notes: a Not including doctors with previous qualifications b Jan. 1984 graduate
c Jan. 1984 graduate
Source: Parkhouse and Parkhouse 1989b

The 1977 qualifiers

1 There were 3,112 students from UK medical schools who obtained university degrees qualifying them to practise medicine in 1977. This figure includes Cambridge graduates who passed both MB and BCh examinations in 1977 and received the BCh degree in that year, even though the MB degree was not conferred until 1978. The number also includes one doctor who obtained qualifying medical degrees from both Cambridge and the University of Wales.

2 There were 85 students from UK medical schools who obtained a non-university qualifying examination in medicine in 1977 and who did not also obtain in that year, and had not previously obtained, a qualifying university degree in medicine.

3 Of this total of 3,197 doctors obtaining a university *or* a non-university qualification in 1977 there were 38 who had already become eligible to practise medicine in previous years, by passing non-university qualifying examinations in 1976 or earlier, and in one case forty-eight years previously. These doctors were not included in our survey of 1977 qualifiers; by the beginning of 1977 they were either already registered with the GMC, or abroad, or not practising medicine.

4 There were thus 3,159 doctors from UK medical schools who became eligible to register with the GMC for the first time in 1977.

5 Twelve of the doctors who qualified for the first time in 1977 from UK medical schools appear never to have registered with the GMC. Seven of these can be guessed from their names to be British, and five are likely to be foreign. One 1977 qualifier died in 1977 and another in 1978.

6 We compiled our list of 1977 qualifiers, for our survey, from the GMC fortnightly lists. This comprised 3,139 doctors, including one doctor who actually graduated in 1976 and was incorrectly shown on registration with the GMC as a 1977 qualifier.

We therefore missed twenty-one people who obtained primary medical qualifications for the first time in 1977. As well as the twelve who never registered with the GMC there were three who did not register until 1979 or 1980; one of these doctors then obtained provisional registration and two obtained full registration without having been provisionally registered, presumably having completed the equivalent of a pre-registration year abroad. The remaining six doctors did obtain provisional registration in 1977 and it therefore seems that we missed them for some unknown reason.

7 A total of 262 doctors obtained *both* university and non-university qualifying examinations in 1977. Of these, 248 were from London medical schools. Thirteen were from English provincial schools, one from Wales and none from the Scottish medical schools. It is interesting to note that the numbers of students taking both examinations varied widely between medical schools — ranging from nil to seventy-one in the London schools and nil to seven in the English provincial schools.

Of the eighty-five doctors who obtained only a non-university medical qualification in 1977, twenty-eight obtained university qualifying degrees in medicine in 1978, and a further four had obtained such degrees by 1980.

8 Of the seventy-nine Oxford University BM BCh graduates in 1977, sixty-two were clinical medical students at Oxford (including one not on our survey list) and seventeen were at London medical schools. Of 167 Cambridge University MB BCh graduates in 1977, 159 were clinical undergraduates at London medical schools; two were at Newcastle, one at Wales, and three at Cambridge, including two who had already qualified MRCS LRCP in 1976. The clinical schools of the two Cambridge graduates who never registered with the GMC were not identified by us.

One London university graduate was a clinical undergraduate student at Bristol, all the rest being at London medical schools except for one student at Liverpool who had already qualified MRCS LRCP in 1976. Of the 1,158 doctors we identified as qualifying in medicine from London medical schools, 918 obtained a London university MB BS, 159 obtained a Cambridge MB BCh, 17 obtained an Oxford BM BCh and 64 obtained a non-university qualification.

The 1983 qualifiers

The situation in 1983 was further complicated by the fact that the London university students who passed the MB BS examinations in December 1982 were awarded their degrees in January 1983. They are therefore 1983 qualifiers, although they actually belonged to the class of 1982. Similarly the 127 members of the 1983 class who passed the MB BS in December 1983 were not awarded their degrees until January 1984, and are therefore registered as 1984 qualifiers. For our survey of '1983 qualifiers' we included all these doctors and thus over-estimated the number who actually *graduated* in the calendar year 1983 by 127. Table 2.5 shows figures with and without the January 1984 London University graduates. The following notes refer only the qualifiers of the calendar year 1983.

1 There were 3,729 students from UK medical schools who obtained university qualifying degrees.
2 There were 41 students who obtained one or more non-university qualifying examinations in medicine and did not also obtain in 1983, and had not previously obtained, a qualifying university degree in medicine.
3 Of this total 3,770 doctors obtaining a university *or* a non-university qualification, there were 27 who had previously passed non-university qualifying examinations and were therefore not included in our survey of 1983 qualifiers.
4 There were thus 3,743 doctors from UK medical schools who became eligible to register with the GMC for the first time in 1983.
5 Five of the doctors who qualified for the first time in 1983 from UK medical schools appear never to have registered with the GMC. Judging from names and available addresses, four of these are foreign and one is likely to be British. They were not included in our survey list.
6 Three other doctors were missing from our survey list. Two of these never proceeded beyond provisional registration and one was not registered by 1984.
7 Our survey list of 1983 qualifiers therefore included 3,735 names, eight fewer than the identified number of first-time qualifiers.
8 There were eighteen doctors who obtained *both* university and non-university qualifying examinations in 1983. Of these, nine were from London medical schools, seven from Oxford and Cambridge and two from other English provincial medical schools.

  Among the 127 London students who graduated in January 1984, there were 16 who had already obtained non-university qualifications in 1983. By 1987, three more of the doctors who obtained only non-university qualifications in 1983 had registered subsequent university qualifying degrees in medicine.
9 Of 128 Cambridge MB BCh graduates in 1983, 81 were clinical students in Cambridge, 41 in London and 1 in Leeds. The clinical medical schools of five Cambridge graduates who had obtained non-university qualifications before 1983

were not identified by us.

All 86 Oxford BM BCh graduates were clinical students at Oxford.

All of the London university graduates were clinical students at London teaching hospitals. Of 1,354 qualifiers from London teaching hospitals, 1,285 were London University graduates, 41 were Cambridge graduates and 28 obtained only non-university qualifications.

The general conclusion to be drawn from this analysis is that the lists which we compiled for our calendar-year surveys of qualifiers from medical schools in the UK were fairly close to the true numbers of people becoming eligible to practise medicine for the first time in the years concerned. The most striking changes that had taken place between 1977 and 1983 were in the very much smaller numbers of students sitting non-university qualifying examinations as well as taking a degree. The traditions and the prevailing advice about taking Conjoint as an insurance policy in case of failure in the MB BS, which had obviously been predominantly a London phenomenon with wide variations between one medical school and another, had altered profoundly: failure rates in the final university examination were low, and taking extra examinations was becoming an increasingly expensive business. Also, by 1983 the Cambridge clinical school was taking an appreciable number of students, and the policy in Oxford had altered so that the Oxford BM BCh degree was reserved for students who had remained in Oxford for the clinical part of the course whereas previously Oxford pre-clinical students who completed the course in London or other medical schools were permitted to sit the Oxford final examination.

A significant finding is that of all the students who qualified in medicine from UK medical schools, including foreign-based students, the number who did not at least provisionally register with the GMC was extremely small.

SURVEY METHODS

For 1974 qualifiers we originally obtained names and addresses from the individual medical schools. We received generous co-operation but compiling complete information was time-consuming and involved a personal visit in one case to copy out lists by hand. For subsequent surveys we relied on the GMC fortnightly lists, following these well into the subsequent year in order to pick up people who may have qualified late in the year and who sometimes did not register until the spring. For 1983 qualifiers, we also obtained from the GMC copies of the certified lists of university and non-university qualifiers.

Apart from one or two early surveys, questionnaires at two-yearly intervals have always been sent to *all* identified qualifiers of the years concerned, at home and abroad, whenever any kind of address was available, regardless of whether a previous response had ever been obtained. The only exceptions were doctors who had specifically asked not to be written to again. In this way we continued to pick up new respondents as the years went by. Questionnaires sent to doctors who had not replied regularly included a supplement, requesting background information and retrospective data on jobs and postgraduate qualifications. We discovered occasional errors, that is, doctors who should not have been included in the surveys. In various ways, over the years, we also found a small number of doctors who had been missed from our original lists and who were then written to. Thus the numbers referred to in Tables 2.2 to 2.5, and the base figures for the numbers of doctors in each of our main cohorts relate to the latest, amended survey lists.

Questionnaires were mailed in the spring of each year, with a reply-paid envelope. This was the time when most qualifiers were three-quarters of the way through the pre-registration year, and had had some time to think about their future plans. It also gave time for a first reminder to be sent to non-respondents before a massive change of addresses took place in midsummer. In fact, two reminders were always sent, the second going to an alternative address if one could be found. The Medical Register and the Medical Directory were searched for addresses, and we owe gratitude to the Medical Mailing Company for supplying print-outs free of charge, which were often most valuable. Some addresses were found from foreign medical registers and directories and we had help on several occasions from respondents who had themselves compiled lists for reunions. For doctors who could still not be traced, or from whom we had not heard after the second reminder, we sought help from the General Medical Council, who were unfailingly co-operative and were often able to supply different addresses. Altogether, the exercise begun in the spring invariably ran on into the following year, at which time late replies were still continuing to arrive. On more than one occasion we received the questionnaire sent two years previously!

Questionnaires were sometimes filled in and returned by parents or others on behalf of doctors working abroad. From these contacts we could often obtain an address and hence a direct reply; otherwise, factual information given about the doctor, such as marital status and location, was recorded if recent enough to be reliable, but opinions such as intentions regarding permanent emigration and reasons for this were not recorded. Gaps or discrepancies in information were occasionally sorted out by personal contact with individual respondents.

The wording of questions and the choice of options, for example of reasons for career choice, were made as unambiguous as possible, at the risk of over-simplification. For the actual specifying of career choices, respondents were asked to indicate three choices in order of preference with the option of bracketing two or three choices as equally desirable. In the first questionnaire, to 1974 qualifiers in 1975, the preamble to this question stated:

> You may be as specific as you like about your career preferences — for instance, if you are determined to be a paediatric neurologist or a cardiac surgeon. If it is more appropriate for you to express your preferences in broad terms, it would help us if you would use the 'mainstream' headings [as in the Todd Report, see p. 8]. To these you may, of course, add academic work, medical work in the armed forces, mission work overseas, etc., etc.

The attempt to classify preferences according to mainstreams did not prove more helpful than giving free rein to respondents. The next questionnaire, to 1975 qualifiers in 1976, stated:

> Be as specific or as general as you like — for instance, paediatric cardiology, mission work abroad, general practice with hospital sessions, etc.

The risk of putting ideas into people's minds became clear when no fewer than 12.1 per cent of respondents gave their first choice as general practice with hospital sessions. From then onwards we abandoned all examples or other potential leads as being much more likely to do harm than good; the subsequent questionnaires were worded:

> List up to three choices of career in order of preference. Bracket any choices that are equal. You can be as specific or as general as you like.

All replies were treated as strictly confidential, as stated in the covering letters accompanying questionnaires. No personally identifiable information has been released to others beyond the project team, or used for other purposes.

DATA MANAGEMENT

Questionnaires were designed to facilitate coding, and all information other than free comment was dealt with by an extensive coding scheme devised for the purpose. This included, for example, eighty-six separate codes for specialties and other occupations, with sub-specialty codes to indicate special interests, academic posts, private sector or armed forces employment, etc. For each respondent in the four main cohorts of 1974, 1977, 1980 and 1983 qualifiers, the data from each questionnaire reply were transferred to a master sheet, which thus provided a complete record of the doctor's preferences and progress through the years in so far as they had been voluntarily supplied to us. Occasional obvious omissions were added after checking with the Medical Directory, for example a senior registrar or consultant in medicine who had not mentioned that he held the MRCP. Data from the master sheets, along with coded data from all individual questionnaires, were punched and entered on to computer files for analysis, mainly using software packages SPSS(X). In compiling master sheets, data punching, checking master sheets against questionnaires, and analysing computer output, opportunities for verification and picking up of errors arose at various stages. Code numbers were assigned to all doctors in the surveys. For each respondent in the 1974, 1977, 1980 and 1983 cohorts there was thus a set of original questionnaires, a named and code-numbered master sheet including all information from the questionnaires except personal comments, and a code-numbered computer tape entry including all information from the master sheet except the name.

Career choices were corrected for ties. The decision to do this was taken during the early Sheffield/Manchester studies. Although there is some air of artificiality about saying that there were 0.3 first choices for endocrinology or that two and a half people apparently wanted to do something else, the system gives a much fairer representation of the relative popularity of different options than any reasonable alternative. If two career options were bracketed by a respondent as equal first choices, each was counted as half a choice; if three were bracketed as equal, each was counted as a third of a choice. Difficulties arise over changes of choice because of the complexity of dealing with a large number of specialties when there are almost unrestricted

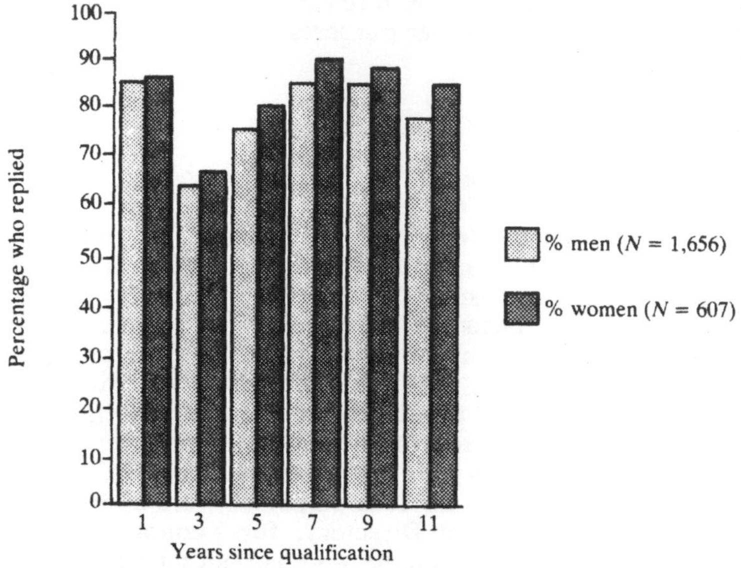

Figure 2.1 Response rates (1974 respondents)
Source: Adapted from Rhodes 1989a

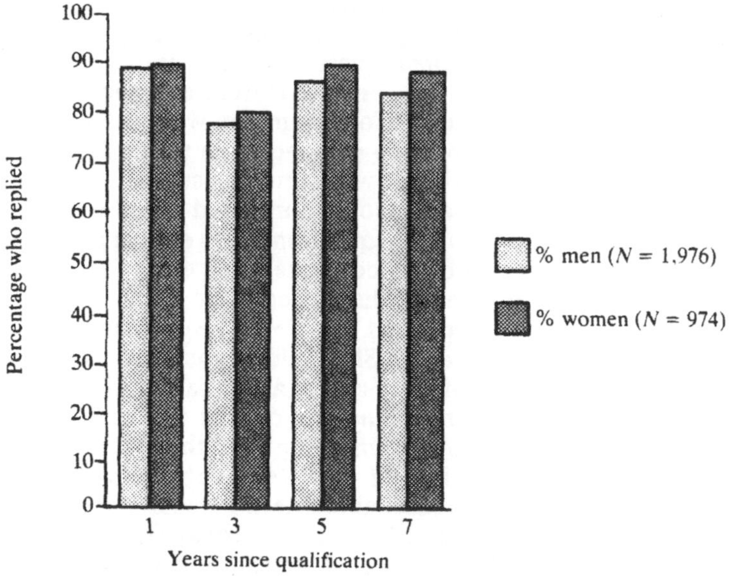

Figure 2.2 Response rates (1977 respondents)
Source: Adapted from Rhodes 1989a

possibilities for changing from one to any other in the early years after qualifying. Also, it is not possible to use tie-corrected *choices* to show the numbers of *people* who have changed their choice: it is simply necessary to decide whether individuals who have changed their choice from medicine bracketed with general practice to general practice alone have changed their choice of specialty, or their firmness of intent. These questions are dealt with in the next chapter.

RESPONSE RATES

The great advantage of a longitudinal study, extending over many years, is that data can be augmented and revised continually as new information comes in. This does create some problems, however, in defining the population base and in reporting percentages of respondents for various purposes.

Response rates for individual surveys can be calculated from the number of questionnaires sent and the number returned by the time results are analysed; these are shown in Table 2.1. There were always some questionnaires sent back 'gone away' and no alternative address was found. A few doctors wrote declining to participate and a few died during the years of the study. Allowing for these factors, our experience was that when we succeeded in getting a questionnaire to a living doctor the level of co-operation was extremely high. Because of the inclusion of late replies, and other amendments described on p. 25, the eventual response rates differ somewhat from those published, and from those shown in Table 2.1.

Figures 2.1 and 2.2 show what percentages of all respondents replied to individual surveys (Rhodes 1989a). They demonstrate the fact that rather higher proportions of women than men responded throughout.

Among individual medical schools, response rates to the initial, pre-registration surveys ranged from 73 per cent to 100 per cent with no consistent pattern. For our four main cohorts (1974, 1977, 1980 and 1983) only seven medical school response rates out of sixty-nine (grouping London medical schools together) were below 80 per cent.

About half the respondents in our studies replied to every questionnaire sent to them and many failed to reply on only one or two occasions. At each survey, up-to-date information was not obtained about some doctors, while valuable retrospective information was obtained from others who had not previously replied for some time, or not at all. By piecing all this information together, and adding in data from late replies, it proved possible for us to obtain some career information for over 95 per cent of each main cohort, and most of this was fairly complete.

Most of the analyses in this book are based on data compiled on to master sheets. For this reason we use the term 'respondent' to define doctors who replied to one or more of the questionnaires sent to them. For example, the statement that 10.3 per cent of 1974 respondents were known to hold the FRCS signifies 10.3 per cent of those 1974 qualifiers who had replied to us at least once and for whom we had some career information. When responses to individual questionnaires are analysed this is noted in the text. There were 2,272 respondents who qualified in 1974 and 2,988 who qualified in 1977: 97.8 and 95.3 per cent of the numbers of doctors in the respective survey populations at their latest revision, that is the numbers of doctors written to in 1987 and 1986 respectively plus those known to have died or not wishing to participate. The corresponding base figures for the numbers of respondents who qualified in 1980 and 1983 were 3,196 (93.5 per cent) and 3,439 (89.5 per cent).

RESULTS

A good deal of information from our research has been published over the years, and the relevant papers are indicated in the Bibliography. By no means all the potentially interesting or useful information has been extracted and analysed from the great mass of data we have obtained. It would take some years to explore every facet, and meanwhile many details would no doubt become out of date and irrelevant. Our aim has been to try and concentrate on the main topics and the quickest reporting that is compatible with reasonable accuracy.

This book gathers together such information as we have to date. Having described the way the studies were done, findings are first presented on career choice, including changes of choice with time, and reasons for these. The next chapters deal with aspects of career progress: examinations, movement of doctors, and the employment position of our respondents at various stages. There are then chapters on individual groups of respondents: women doctors, and those choosing certain specialties which we have looked at in detail. Finally, a chapter deals with comments from respondents, including questionnaire replies on opinions about various aspects of training and competence, and the discussions which took place at the White Hart.

3 Career choice

We have published reports of the career choices of successive cohorts of qualifiers (see Bibliography). We are now able to gather together the information provided by all of our respondents.

CHOICE OF CAREER AT THE PRE-REGISTRATION STAGE

Table 3.1 shows a breakdown of first choices of career, corrected for ties, by 'mainstreams', that is 'medicine' includes the medical specialties, (excepting paediatrics, which is shown separately), and 'surgery' includes the surgical specialties. In this table and Tables 3.2 and 3.3 haematology is included in the pathology mainstream, except that in some of our earlier coding clinical haematology, where mentioned, was separately identified and included within the medicine mainstream. This applied to only a small number of choices.

By far the most popular choice of career throughout was general practice, followed by medicine and surgery. There was a tendency for the popularity of general practice as a first choice to increase from 1974 to 1980, with a very marked jump in popularity between 1980 and 1983, particularly among women respondents. Correspondingly the popularity of medicine and surgery declined over the years; this was particularly notable in the case of medicine and the medical specialties, which accounted for scarcely more than half as many preferences in 1983 as they had done in 1974. Pathology showed a progressive rise in popularity, from 2.8 per cent of first choices among 1974 respondents in 1975 to 4.5 per cent among 1983 respondents in 1984. The popularity of radiology also increased by a comparable order of magnitude. There were few choices for community medicine, although small peaks of interest occurred among 1975 and 1983 qualifiers. Paediatrics showed some decline in popularity over the years studied, with rather more loss of interest among women than among men.

Table 3.1 First career choices: percentages of respondents in the pre-registration year

Specialty		*Year of qualifying* 1974	1975	1976	1977	1978	1979	1980	1983
Medicine	Men	24.8	21.5	21.7	22.7	22.3	20.6	19.0	15.2
	Women	19.3	15.1	17.2	17.3	18.8	17.1	16.9	10.9
	Total	23.2	19.6	20.2	20.9	21.1	19.4	18.2	13.5
Paediatrics	Men	5.0	4.2	5.2	4.2	3.6	2.9	3.1	3.6
	Women	10.4	11.8	9.5	9.0	9.7	6.7	7.4	5.2
	Total	6.6	6.4	6.6	5.8	5.6	4.2	4.6	4.2
Surgery	Men	20.6	19.5	20.8	22.9	22.1	21.3	20.9	17.6
	Women	4.1	5.2	6.4	6.2	5.4	6.4	6.8	4.4
	Total	16.2	15.4	16.2	17.4	16.5	16.1	15.9	12.4
Obstetrics & gynaecology	Men	3.9	3.2	3.4	2.5	2.2	2.2	3.4	2.7
	Women	3.9	3.6	4.7	3.8	6.0	3.2	3.9	4.2
	Total	3.9	3.3	3.8	2.9	3.5	2.5	3.6	3.3
Anaesthetics	Men	4.3	3.3	5.3	4.8	5.6	5.2	5.6	4.6
	Women	4.5	4.8	7.3	6.3	4.7	6.9	6.7	4.7
	Total	4.3	3.8	6.0	5.3	5.3	5.8	6.0	4.6
Pathology	Men	2.2	2.0	2.9	2.9	2.9	3.4	3.4	4.4
	Women	4.2	2.6	4.1	3.9	4.6	4.8	4.4	4.6
	Total	2.8	2.2	3.3	3.2	3.4	3.9	3.8	4.5
Psychiatry	Men	3.4	3.2	2.6	2.9	3.0	3.7	3.4	3.8
	Women	4.0	3.4	3.5	5.4	2.8	4.6	3.3	4.6
	Total	3.6	3.2	2.9	3.7	3.0	4.0	3.4	4.1
Radiology	Men	1.3	1.0	1.6	1.0	1.6	1.3	2.0	2.2
	Women	1.3	1.5	2.4	2.1	3.2	2.5	2.8	2.1
	Total	1.3	1.2	1.8	1.4	2.1	1.7	2.3	2.2
Radiotherapy	Men	0.4	0.6	1.4	0.8	0.8	0.8	1.0	1.2
	Women	1.9	1.4	2.0	1.2	1.1	1.2	1.5	0.8
	Total	0.8	0.8	1.6	0.9	0.9	0.9	1.2	1.1
General practice	Men	30.6	33.4	30.0	30.4	31.5	33.9	34.1	39.5
	Women	41.3	40.7	37.2	39.3	40.4	42.2	41.5	52.5
	Total	33.4	35.5	32.3	33.3	34.5	36.8	36.8	44.7
Community medicine	Men	0.3	1.1	0.5	0.4	0.4	0.4	0.5	1.2
	Women	1.8	2.4	2.0	2.2	1.3	1.6	1.3	2.2
	Total	0.8	1.4	1.0	1.0	0.7	0.8	0.8	1.6
Other medical	Men	1.9	5.5	2.5	2.6	2.2	2.6	2.0	1.8
	Women	2.4	5.4	1.8	1.2	1.1	1.6	1.7	1.6
	Total	2.0	5.5	2.3	2.1	1.8	2.3	1.9	1.8

Table 3.1 continued

Specialty		*Year of qualifying* 1974	1975	1976	1977	1978	1979	1980	1983
Non-medical	Men	0.4	0.6	0.3	0.6	0.5	0.6	0.3	0.6
	Women	0.5	0.8	0.2	0.9	0.1	0.6	0.5	0.8
	Total	0.4	0.6	0.3	0.7	0.4	0.6	0.4	0.7
No career choice		0.7	1.0	1.8	1.3	1.1	0.9	1.2	1.3

Table 3.2 shows second choices of career at the pre-registration stage, again corrected for ties. The table also shows that whereas virtually all respondents indicated a first choice of career, substantial numbers did not give a second choice. Among those who did, there was a decline in the popularity of medicine and surgery, and a relatively greater decline in choices for obstetrics and gynaecology. The rising popularity of general practice as a first choice was to some extent mirrored by less popularity as a second choice.

Table 3.3 shows third choices of career, corrected for ties. Many respondents did not indicate a third choice of career; among those who did, there was a decline in the number of preferences, over the years studied, for general practice, paediatrics, obstetrics and gynaecology, and anaesthetics.

Sex differences

Higher proportions of women than men gave general practice as a first choice of career throughout the years surveyed, the sex difference being greatest in 1983. Similarly paediatrics was very much more commonly given as a first choice by women than men. To a lesser extent the same preponderance of female choices was seen in the other mainstreams, with the exception of medicine and surgery. The preponderance of male choices for surgery and the surgical specialties was overwhelming, with little indication of any real change between 1974 and 1983.

Table 3.2 Second career choices: percentages of respondents in the pre-registration year

		Year of qualifying							
Specialty		*1974*	*1975*	*1976*	*1977*	*1978*	*1979*	*1980*	*1983*
Medicine	Men	21.3	19.2	19.4	19.8	19.1	18.3	17.8	15.7
	Women	18.6	15.5	16.5	19.0	18.9	17.4	15.9	11.6
	Total	20.6	18.1	18.4	19.6	19.0	18.0	17.1	14.1
Paediatrics	Men	5.8	5.4	5.9	5.3	5.2	3.6	4.2	3.5
	Women	10.0	11.1	11.9	9.2	9.7	8.4	7.5	5.0
	Total	6.9	7.1	7.9	6.6	6.7	5.3	5.3	4.1
Surgery	Men	14.2	12.3	12.1	12.8	12.4	12.5	11.1	10.8
	Women	3.4	3.5	4.7	4.6	3.4	3.5	2.6	3.7
	Total	11.2	9.7	9.7	10.1	9.4	9.4	8.1	8.0
Obstetrics &	Men	5.0	2.8	3.2	4.0	3.8	2.2	4.0	2.3
gynaecology	Women	7.0	5.3	5.8	5.2	4.2	4.1	4.0	3.9
	Total	5.6	3.5	4.1	4.4	4.0	2.9	4.0	2.9
Anaesthetics	Men	3.8	4.7	4.2	5.1	5.6	4.8	5.1	3.3
	Women	5.5	4.7	4.7	5.1	4.6	5.0	4.3	3.0
	Total	4.2	4.7	4.4	5.1	5.2	4.9	4.8	3.2
Pathology	Men	3.3	2.1	2.7	3.5	2.5	3.0	3.4	2.5
	Women	3.0	2.7	2.9	4.2	4.4	4.1	4.2	3.9
	Total	3.2	2.2	2.8	3.8	3.2	3.4	3.7	3.1
Psychiatry	Men	3.5	2.3	2.1	3.0	1.9	2.2	2.7	2.9
	Women	4.2	3.9	3.2	3.2	2.1	3.8	3.6	4.8
	Total	3.7	2.7	2.4	3.0	2.0	2.7	3.0	3.7
Radiology	Men	1.7	1.1	1.7	2.3	1.9	2.1	2.5	2.3
	Women	1.2	1.3	1.7	1.5	2.9	2.3	2.5	2.0
	Total	1.6	1.1	1.7	2.0	2.3	2.2	2.5	2.2
Radiotherapy	Men	0.7	0.8	1.2	1.0	0.9	0.8	1.1	1.0
	Women	0.9	1.2	1.1	1.5	1.7	1.0	1.1	1.1
	Total	0.8	0.9	1.1	1.2	1.2	0.9	1.1	1.0
General	Men	18.4	18.6	17.2	17.1	16.2	17.7	12.9	13.5
practice	Women	22.7	21.0	19.8	18.2	19.3	18.5	16.9	15.6
	Total	19.7	19.3	18.0	17.5	17.2	18.0	14.3	14.3
Community	Men	1.4	1.1	1.1	0.8	0.9	0.9	1.2	1.6
medicine	Women	7.8	3.5	1.1	3.1	2.4	3.3	2.2	4.4
	Total	3.1	1.8	1.1	1.6	1.4	1.7	1.5	2.7

Table 3.2 continued

Specialty		*Year of qualifying* 1974	*1975*	*1976*	*1977*	*1978*	*1979*	*1980*	*1983*
Other medical	Men	1.9	3.5	2.4	2.5	2.2	2.4	1.7	2.4
	Women	2.3	6.0	1.4	1.4	1.7	2.3	1.9	2.0
	Total	2.1	4.2	2.1	2.1	2.0	2.3	1.8	2.2
Non-medical	Men	0.3	0.6	0.5	0.6	0.3	0.5	0.2	0.8
	Women	0.5	0.2	0.5	0.2	0.3	0.3	0.4	0.3
	Total	0.3	0.5	0.5	0.5	0.3	0.4	0.3	0.6
No career choice		17.0	24.0	25.9	22.6	26.1	28.0	32.5	37.8

Marital status

Taking the years from 1974 to 1980 inclusive, the career choices of single qualifiers tended to follow the overall patterns shown in the tables, while there was greater variation among married qualifiers. The popularity of paediatrics declined more sharply among married qualifiers than those who were single, but this distinction did not apply in the case of anaesthetics. Obstetrics and gynaecology retained its popularity among single qualifiers, while its popularity fell away among those who were married. Although, overall, psychiatry was equally popular among 1974 and 1980 qualifiers, it was less popular among those who were single and more popular among those who were married in 1980, compared with 1974.

In percentage terms, general practice was the only career choice consistently more popular among married than single qualifiers. In terms of absolute numbers, all specialties were chosen by more single than married respondents.

Pathology and radiology were more popular among married respondents, in five of the seven cohorts from 1974 to 1980 inclusive, and psychiatry in four of the seven. Medicine, paediatrics and surgery were consistently more popular among single qualifiers.

Table 3.3 Third career choices: percentages of respondents in the pre-registration year

		Year of qualifying							
Specialty		*1974*	*1975*	*1976*	*1977*	*1978*	*1979*	*1980*	*1983*
Medicine	Men	7.9	9.3	7.9	10.0	9.1	9.2	7.5	7.6
	Women	10.2	8.2	8.0	8.1	10.4	8.8	7.6	6.1
	Total	8.5	9.0	8.0	9.4	9.6	9.0	7.5	7.0
Paediatrics	Men	3.6	2.5	2.1	3.6	3.0	2.1	2.6	1.4
	Women	6.6	5.3	3.7	4.9	5.4	4.0	3.0	3.3
	Total	7.4	3.3	2.6	4.0	3.8	2.7	2.8	2.2
Surgery	Men	5.8	5.7	5.4	5.6	5.3	5.6	5.4	5.2
	Women	1.2	2.0	2.4	1.9	2.1	1.7	2.0	2.6
	Total	4.5	4.6	4.5	4.3	4.2	4.3	4.2	4.1
Obstetrics & gynaecology	Men	3.2	1.6	2.0	2.1	1.7	1.9	1.3	1.3
	Women	4.7	2.0	3.4	4.2	2.3	3.1	2.0	1.5
	Total	3.6	1.7	2.4	2.8	1.9	2.3	1.5	1.3
Anaesthetics	Men	3.5	2.6	2.9	3.1	3.3	2.4	2.6	1.8
	Women	2.5	2.9	3.4	3.9	2.7	2.7	2.0	1.3
	Total	3.2	2.7	3.0	3.3	3.1	2.5	2.3	1.6
Pathology	Men	2.3	1.7	1.7	2.8	1.9	2.6	1.9	2.4
	Women	2.4	2.8	2.4	2.7	1.9	2.3	3.5	2.5
	Total	2.3	2.0	1.9	2.8	1.9	2.5	2.5	2.4
Psychiatry	Men	2.4	1.9	1.8	1.8	1.5	1.7	1.9	2.4
	Women	3.5	3.1	1.5	2.6	2.5	1.2	1.6	3.1
	Total	2.7	2.3	1.7	2.1	1.8	1.5	1.8	2.7
Radiology	Men	1.4	1.1	1.4	1.6	1.0	1.9	1.5	2.0
	Women	2.8	1.3	1.1	1.8	1.9	1.0	1.1	1.3
	Total	1.7	1.2	1.3	1.7	1.3	1.6	1.4	1.7
Radiotherapy	Men	0.7	0.5	0.7	0.4	0.6	0.4	0.9	0.3
	Women	0.7	0.9	0.5	0.6	0.4	0.2	0.6	0.4
	Total	0.7	0.6	0.7	0.5	0.5	0.3	0.8	0.3
General practice	Men	17.5	13.5	13.2	13.9	13.4	11.7	10.2	8.0
	Women	13.6	12.3	11.3	13.6	11.9	10.9	8.6	6.9
	Total	16.4	13.2	12.6	13.8	12.9	11.4	9.6	7.5
Community medicine	Men	2.2	0.8	0.8	0.7	0.8	0.5	0.9	0.9
	Women	4.7	2.2	1.4	1.4	1.1	2.3	1.7	2.3
	Total	2.9	1.2	1.0	1.0	0.9	1.1	1.2	1.4

Table 3.3 continued

Specialty		*Year of qualifying* 1974	1975	1976	1977	1978	1979	1980	1983
Other medical	Men	1.5	3.0	2.0	1.9	1.4	1.8	1.1	1.4
	Women	0.7	3.4	1.0	1.1	1.0	1.4	1.3	1.3
	Total	1.3	3.1	1.7	1.6	1.3	1.6	1.2	1.4
Non-medical	Men	0.4	0.9	0.9	1.8	0.6	1.5	0.7	0.7
	Women	0.1	0.4	1.0	0.1	0.3	0.9	0.4	0.6
	Total	0.3	0.8	0.9	1.2	0.5	1.3	0.6	0.6
No career choice		47.4	54.3	57.8	51.6	56.3	57.8	62.6	65.6

Mature qualifiers

Over the years 1974-80 inclusive, 8.3-10.8 per cent of respondents were aged 27 or over in the pre-registration year; 13.8-20.5 per cent were 26 or over. For the purposes of arriving at a reasonable definition, we regarded mature qualifiers as those who were aged 27 or over at the time of their reply in the pre-registration year for 1974-79 qualifiers, and 27 or over on 1 April 1981 for 1980 qualifiers. Among 1974 respondents, 42.6 per cent of mature qualifiers had obtained qualifications of some kind before entering medical school, compared to 4.5 per cent of all respondents. Among 1980 qualifiers, 59.3 per cent of mature qualifiers had qualifications before entering medical school, compared to 5.5 per cent of all respondents.

For most specialties, the popularity of first career choices among mature qualifiers during the years 1974-80 followed the general pattern for all qualifiers, but there were some consistent differences worth noting.

Among mature qualifiers general practice, anaesthetics, radiology and radiotherapy did not show the general increase in popularity over the years studied. Psychiatry and community medicine increased in popularity among mature qualifiers; surgery showed a slight rise in popularity from 1978 onwards, compared with its steady fall among respondents in general.

Table 3.4 Firmness of first choice of career in the pre-registration year: percentages of respondents and specialties with highest and lowest proportions of definite choices

Year of qualifying		*Definite*	*Probable*	*Uncertain*	*Most definite*	*Least definite*
1974	Men	28.3	49.6	21.9	Psychiatry	Radiotherapy
	Women	17.3	54.8	27.5	GP	Radiotherapy
	Total	25.1	51.2	23.4	GP	Radiotherapy
1975	Men	24.3	47.5	26.8	Surgery	Radiotherapy
	Women	18.1	48.6	32.2	Anaesthetics	Paediatrics
	Total	22.5	47.8	28.2	Surgery	Radiotherapy
1976	Men	26.5	48.0	24.1	Surgery and GP	Radiotherapy
	Women	17.9	46.8	34.3	Surgery	Non-medical and comm. med.
	Total	23.8	47.6	27.4	Surgery	Community medicine
1977	Men	23.4	50.6	25.0	Radiology	Non-medical
	Women	19.4	49.0	31.1	Surgery	Community medicine
	Total	22.1	50.1	27.0	Surgery	Community medicine
1978	Men	29.2	47.9	21.9	GP	Community medicine
	Women	20.6	54.2	23.6	GP	Non-medical
	Total	26.3	50.0	22.5	GP	Non-medical
1979	Men	34.2	45.8	19.3	GP	Non-medical
	Women	24.6	50.4	24.1	GP	Non-medical and comm. med.
	Total	30.9	47.4	21.0	GP	Non-medical
1980	Men	28.9	48.5	22.4	Psychiatry	Non-medical
	Women	25.1	48.0	26.5	GP	Radiotherapy and other medical
	Total	27.5	48.3	23.9	GP	Non-medical
1983	Men	40.2	46.1	12.8	GP	Non-medical
	Women	35.6	47.7	16.2	GP	Community medicine
	Total	38.3	46.8	14.2	GP	Community medicine

There was a decline in the popularity of paediatrics among mature qualifiers, as for all respondents, and again this decline was more pronounced among women than men. The increasing popularity of pathology was more marked among mature qualifiers, particularly mature women, for whom it was the third most popular choice after general practice and medicine in the

1976, 1977, 1979 and 1980 cohorts. In fact, pathology was consistently more popular among mature qualifiers, and the difference between its popularity among mature qualifiers and all respondents tended to increase during the years surveyed. Paediatrics was the only specialty less popular among mature qualifiers than all respondents in each of the seven years from 1974 to 1980; but radiology and anaesthetics were less popular among mature qualifiers than overall in six of these seven cohorts. Interestingly the same applied to general practice.

Firmness of choice

Table 3.4 shows the proportions of respondents from the various years who regarded their first choices of career at the pre-registration stage as definite, probable, or uncertain, by sex. It also shows the specialties with the highest and lowest proportions of definite career choices.

The most notable points are first the fact that until 1980, only about a quarter of our respondents had made a definite choice of career by the time that most of them were nearing the end of their pre-registration year. Second, there was a marked increase in the proportion of definite choices among 1983 qualifiers, and this is perhaps reflected in the increasing percentages of respondents, in the later years of our surveys, who did not give second or third choices of career (Tables 3.2 and 3.3). Higher proportions of men than women were definite about their career choices throughout our surveys; correspondingly frank uncertainty was more commonly expressed by women than men in every cohort.

In five of the eight years surveyed, general practice was the career with the highest proportion of definite choosers, and surgery showed the highest proportion in the other three years. Among men, psychiatry had the highest number of definite choosers on two occasions. The lowest proportions of definite choosers were found among those opting for community medicine, non-medical careers, and radiotherapy.

Intentions regarding emigration

Table 3.5 shows the way that respondents at the pre-registration stage answered the question about whether, apart from time-limited experiences abroad, they intended eventually to practise in the UK. The proportion of respondents who answered

Table 3.5 Intentions expressed at pre-registration stage regarding practising in the UK: percentages of respondents and specialties with highest and lowest proportions of 'definitely yes' replies

Year of qualifying		*Definitely yes*	*Definitely no*	*Probably yes*	*Probably no*	*Uncertain*	*Most definitely yes*	*Least definitely yes*
1974	Men	29.3	2.8	50.6	8.4	8.7	Psychiatry	Paediatrics
	Women	39.5	1.5	48.5	5.3	5.1	Radiology	Non-medical
	Total	32.0	2.5	50.0	7.5	7.8	Radiology	Non-medical
1975	Men	34.1	2.3	46.6	8.9	7.7	GP	Non-medical
	Women	39.6	1.4	46.7	5.4	6.7	Radiology	Non-medical
	Total	35.7	2.0	46.6	7.9	7.4	GP	Non-medical
1976	Men	31.6	1.9	44.5	9.3	12.6	GP	Non-medical
	Women	39.6	1.7	46.5	4.5	7.5	Non-medical	Other medical
	Total	34.2	1.8	45.1	7.7	10.9	Community medicine	Other medical
1977	Men	30.8	1.6	51.4	6.2	9.6	Psychiatry	Radiology
	Women	38.6	1.0	48.9	4.2	7.1	Community medicine	Non-medical
	Total	33.4	1.4	50.6	5.5	8.8	Community medicine	Non-medical
1978	Men	35.2	1.8	46.8	6.0	9.7	Radiotherapy	Non-medical
	Women	43.8	1.1	45.0	3.8	5.8	Psychiatry	Non-medical
	Total	38.1	1.6	46.2	5.3	8.4	Radiotherapy	Non-medical
1979	Men	41.8	1.4	45.4	5.3	4.0	Community medicine	Non-medical
	Women	48.7	0.9	41.8	4.2	3.0	Psychiatry	Other medical
	Total	44.2	1.2	44.1	4.9	3.6	GP	Non-medical
1980	Men	46.9	1.4	42.2	5.5	3.7	GP	Non-medical
	Women	51.2	0.7	41.7	3.6	2.8	GP	Non-medical
	Total	48.5	1.2	42.0	4.8	3.4	GP	Non-medical
1983	Men	48.7	2.0	39.6	5.1	4.1	GP	Other medical
	Women	48.0	1.4	41.5	4.4	4.2	Radiotherapy	Non-medical
	Total	48.4	1.8	40.3	4.8	4.2	GP	Other medical

'definitely yes' rose fairly steadily, from 32.0 per cent among 1974 respondents in 1975 to 48.4 per cent among 1983 respondents in 1984. At the same time, the proportions answering 'probably no' and 'definitely no' declined. In every cohort except 1983 the proportion of women who answered 'definitely yes' was higher than the proportion of men and, although the numbers were small, the proportions of men who answered 'definitely no' were always higher than those of women. In contrast to the firmness of career choice, the proportions of respondents who were frankly uncertain about their emigration intentions were always slightly higher among men than among women.

Respondents who gave general practice or community medicine as their first choice of career were most likely to intend definitely to remain in the UK. Among the individual cohorts, radiotherapy featured as the specialty choice with the highest proportion of 'definitely yes' responses once for both men and women combined, once for women and once for men; radiology featured twice for women and psychiatry twice for men and twice for women.

Respondents among whom the lowest proportions intended definitely to remain in the UK were those choosing non-medical careers or a variety of medical occupations outside the general run of mainstreams, with paediatrics and radiology each featuring in one cohort among men.

Medical school differences

The tables in this chapter have so far given information for all medical schools combined.

Table 3.6 shows the average percentages of respondents who gave each of the mainstreams as their first choice of career, corrected for ties, at the pre-registration stage for all the years surveyed, by medical school. The table thus makes it possible to form an estimate of whether, over the whole period 1974-80 plus 1983, there was a tendency for qualifiers from some medical schools to show more or fewer preferences for particular specialties than those from other medical schools.

The average proportion of choices for medicine ranged from less than 15 per cent in Leicester, Aberdeen and Dundee to over 25 per cent in two of the London teaching hospitals, St George's and the Westminster. In paediatrics the range of popularity was from less than 3 per cent at Leicester and St George's to over 7 per cent in Belfast, University College Hospital and Manchester. The lowest proportions of choices for surgery: less than 12 per

Table 3.6 First choices of career at the pre-registration stage for main specialty groups: percentages of respondents from all years surveyed[a]

Medical School	*Medicine*	*Paediatrics*	*Surgery*	*Obstetrics & gynaecology*	*Anaesthetics*	*Pathology*	*Psychiatry*	*Radiology*	*Radio-therapy*	*General practice*	*Community medicine*
Aberdeen	12.5---	3.1--	13.3	3.4	7.8+++	3.3	4.7	1.7	0.3	45.6+++	0.8
Dundee	14.0---	4.1	19.1++	4.1	7.1+	3.7	2.5	1.5	0.6	37.2	1.0
Edinburgh	18.3	6.2	14.9	4.9++	7.2++	3.1	4.0	1.0	0.8	34.4	0.8
Glasgow	19.0	4.8	16.4	4.3	5.8	4.8++	4.7++	2.4	0.4	32.4--	1.1
Birmingham	16.6-	5.6	15.4	1.1---	4.7	2.9	4.6	1.4	1.1	40.6++	1.3
Bristol	15.8--	5.4	11.9--	1.9-	5.3	3.8	4.0	1.8	1.4	41.5+++	1.8++
Cambridge	20.3	5.0	23.1+++	3.7	1.7--	4.1	3.7	1.7	2.1	28.3--	1.0
Leeds	16.1-	4.5	13.6	2.6	6.4	2.1-	4.0	1.0	1.0	44.0+++	0.7
Leicester	9.9--	2.2	14.7	5.2	5.2	3.4	8.2++	0.9	0.4	44.7	1.1
Liverpool	18.9	5.6	16.4	5.4+++	6.4	2.4	3.4	2.6	0.5	33.9	0.8
Manchester	18.1	8.6+++	14.5	3.5	3.9-	2.0--	2.7	1.4	1.1	38.7+	1.2
Newcastle	16.8	5.1	13.3	3.3	5.5	3.7	3.7	2.1	0.8	40.5++	1.3
Nottingham	16.0	5.8	9.7--	2.9	4.7	3.4	4.5	2.9	1.1	44.0++	2.0
Oxford	24.2++	5.4	16.6	1.1--	4.1	5.0	3.5	1.5	1.4	30.3--	1.8
Sheffield	16.1-	6.2	13.0-	3.0	4.5	4.3	2.5	1.8	1.0	44.2+++	0.3
Southampton	19.7	5.8	14.8	2.1	5.2	4.3	3.3	1.1	1.2	37.8	0.9

Table 3.6 continued

Medical School	*Medicine*	*Paediatrics*	*Surgery*	*Obstetrics & gynaecology*	*Anaesthetics*	*Pathology*	*Psychiatry*	*Radiology*	*Radio-therapy*	*General practice*	*Community medicine*
Charing Cross	19.5	4.2	18.4	2.6	5.1	2.8	1.9-	0.8	1.5	37.4	1.4
Guy's	21.8	4.7	18.0	3.0	3.4	3.5	3.6	1.5	0.4	35.7	0.3-
King's College	21.9	4.8	14.9	4.6	6.0	3.4	3.2	2.2	0.8	33.3	0.6
The London	19.9	5.8	19.3++	2.4	4.4	3.0	2.8	1.0	0.6	35.6	0.8
Middlesex	22.8++	5.5	18.7+	2.3	2.4---	4.2	3.4	0.8	2.7	31.9--	1.2
Royal Free	19.2	5.0	13.3	3.6	2.7--	4.6	2.3	1.7	1.8	41.4++	0.6
St Bart's	17.8	3.9	19.7+++	4.0	6.3	3.1	3.8	2.3	2.5	29.2---	1.2
St George's	26.4+++	2.9-	16.8	2.8	3.5	3.3	7.2+++	1.6	0.7	31.1-	0.2
St Mary's	23.1++	4.7	14.2	3.1	4.7	2.8	3.0	1.8	0.9	35.8	1.6
St Thomas'	24.4+++	4.9	21.7+++	4.3	6.6	4.9	1.4--	1.9	0.5	25.2---	0.7
UCH	23.8++	7.5++	13.9	2.5	4.4	3.9	4.3	1.0	1.6	30.8--	1.0
Westminster	28.0+++	4.7	18.3	2.6	4.0	2.0	1.9	1.8	2.6	29.3---	0.5
Wales	22.4+	5.0	13.7	3.8	5.6	3.1	2.5	4.4	0.2	34.9	1.3
Belfast	18.0	7.2+	12.6-	4.7+	6.7	4.9+	3.9	2.7	0.7	35.8	0.9

Note: a High or low probability of a specialty being chosen among respondents with career choices from a medical school, compared to the overall probability of the specialty being chosen, among all respondents with career choices, is indicated: z statistic significant at 5% + or -; 1% ++ or --; 0.1% +++ or ---

Table 3.7 First choices of career at the pre-registration stage for medical specialties: percentages of respondents from all years surveyed

Medical school	*Cardiology*	*Dermatology*	*Endo-crinology*	*Geriatrics*	*Haematology*	*Nephrology*	*Neurology*	*Rheumatology*	*Thoracic medicine*	*All specialties shown*
Aberdeen	0.00	0.29	0.00	0.19	0.07	0.00	0.65	0.00	0.14	1.34
Dundee	0.30	0.48	0.15	0.52	0.86	0.00	0.19	0.15	0.15	2.80
Edinburgh	0.61	0.31	0.20	0.36	1.10	0.31	0.31	0.05	0.16	3.41
Glasgow	0.53	0.86	0.00	0.31	2.30	0.23	0.11	0.00	0.08	4.42
Birmingham	0.51	0.20	0.13	0.00	0.51	0.10	0.20	0.10	0.00	1.75
Bristol	0.34	0.55	0.40	0.89	1.20	0.06	0.96	0.16	0.06	4.62
Cambridge	1.40	0.21	0.43	0.68	0.98	0.00	1.49	0.43	0.43	6.05
Leeds	0.39	0.91	0.13	0.04	0.71	0.04	0.00	0.52	0.13	2.87
Leicester	0.00	0.00	0.00	0.00	1.72	0.00	0.00	0.00	0.00	1.72
Liverpool	0.17	0.80	0.23	0.11	1.12	0.00	0.63	0.06	0.46	3.58
Manchester	0.43	0.81	0.00	0.30	0.40	0.09	0.67	0.13	0.13	2.96
Newcastle	0.36	0.58	0.19	1.17	0.84	0.04	0.75	0.06	0.17	4.16
Nottingham	0.29	0.29	0.29	0.66	0.43	0.00	0.94	0.00	0.00	2.90
Oxford	1.36	0.59	0.35	0.23	0.86	0.54	1.13	0.38	0.23	5.70
Sheffield	0.42	1.08	0.00	0.49	0.83	0.00	0.32	0.00	0.07	3.21
Southampton	0.23	1.82	0.00	0.42	0.23	0.23	0.70	0.12	0.23	3.98

Table 3.7 continued

Medical school	*Cardiology*	*Dermatology*	*Endo-crinology*	*Geriatrics*	*Haematology*	*Nephrology*	*Neurology*	*Rheumatology*	*Thoracic medicine*	*All specialties shown*
Charing Cross	0.19	0.09	0.09	0.37	0.06	0.19	1.03	0.37	0.19	2.58
Guy's	0.61	0.90	0.38	0.51	0.92	0.23	0.88	0.38	0.42	5.23
King's College	1.18	0.21	0.16	0.24	0.69	0.16	1.30	0.61	0.32	4.87
The London	0.27	0.27	0.00	0.14	1.02	0.14	0.61	0.27	0.00	2.72
Middlesex	0.76	0.87	0.90	0.28	0.80	0.48	0.53	0.69	0.14	5.45
Royal Free	0.48	0.85	0.16	0.37	1.00	0.00	1.05	0.48	0.64	5.03
St Bart's	0.69	0.96	0.25	0.06	0.47	0.37	0.47	0.71	0.37	4.35
St George's	0.69	0.37	0.00	0.37	0.94	0.00	0.57	0.12	0.86	3.92
St Mary's	0.76	0.47	0.15	0.15	0.64	0.15	0.61	0.27	0.92	4.12
St Thomas'	0.78	0.83	0.00	0.17	1.04	0.00	0.63	0.17	0.05	3.67
UCH	0.50	0.61	0.90	0.29	1.59	0.21	1.26	0.21	0.00	5.57
Westminster	0.82	0.82	0.52	0.58	0.82	0.00	0.82	0.47	0.27	5.12
Wales	0.73	0.50	0.13	0.23	1.07	0.00	0.25	0.23	0.54	3.68
Belfast	0.33	0.59	0.00	0.65	0.52	0.00	0.00	0.00	0.00	2.09

cent came from Nottingham and Bristol, while the highest (over 20 per cent) were from St Thomas' Hospital and Cambridge. An average of more than 5 per cent of respondents chose obstetrics and gynaecology from Liverpool and Leicester, and less than 2 per cent from Bristol, Birmingham and Oxford. In anaesthetics the range was from less than 3 per cent at Cambridge, the Middlesex Hospital, and the Royal Free Hospital, to over 7 per cent in three of the four Scottish medical schools — Aberdeen, Dundee and Edinburgh. Pathology featured most prominently among qualifiers from Oxford, Glasgow, St Thomas', the Royal Free Hospital and Belfast, and least frequently among those from the Westminster Hospital, Liverpool, Leeds and Manchester. Outstandingly the highest average proportion of choices for psychiatry came from Leicester (8.2 per cent) and St George's Hospital (7.2 per cent). Other medical schools which produced an average of between 4.5 and 5.0 per cent of first choices for psychiatry were Aberdeen, Glasgow and Birmingham, while less than 2 per cent came from Charing Cross, the Westminster, and St Thomas'. The University of Wales College of Medicine produced an average of 4.4 per cent first choices for radiology — substantially higher than any other medical school. The next highest figures were from Nottingham, Belfast and Liverpool, with the lowest figures (less than 1 per cent) being from Leicester, Middlesex Hospital and Charing Cross Hospital. Average choices for radiotherapy ranged from 2.7 and 2.6 per cent at Middlesex Hospital and Westminster Hospital to 0.3 per cent at Aberdeen and 0.2 per cent in Wales. The medical schools which produced an average of more than 1.5 per cent of first choices for community medicine were Nottingham, Bristol, Oxford and St Mary's Hospital.

Some of the largest differences between medical schools were in the average numbers of first choices for general practice. These ranged from over 40 per cent of respondents in nine medical schools (45.6 per cent from Aberdeen) to less than 30 per cent in four medical schools (25.2 per cent from St Thomas' Hospital). The average exceeded 40 per cent in only one of the London teaching hospitals, and was below 30 per cent in three.

All of the figures in Tables 3.6, 3.7 and 3.8 relate to the *clinical* medical school of the qualifiers concerned. Thus, the figures for Cambridge refer only to those qualifiers who remained in Cambridge for the clinical part of the course. Clinical students from Oxford and Cambridge who, for example, undertook the clinical part of their course in a London teaching hospital are included with the figures for that London teaching hospital. It should be noted that the Leicester medical school produced its first graduates in 1980, so the average percentages of first choices for that medical school are based on two cohorts only. This makes the percentage of choices for medicine (9.9) less surprising in view of the fact that by 1980 the general popularity of medicine had declined considerably (Table 3.1).

Looking across the figures generally, there is a tendency for a lower number of preferences for general practice to be associated with a high popularity of medicine and the medical specialties, pathology, and perhaps surgery and the surgical specialties. This pattern is seen among the qualifiers from Cambridge, Oxford, Middlesex Hospital, St Thomas' Hospital, and University College Hospital.

Table 3.7 displays similar information for the medical specialties. The percentages of first choices, being small, are shown to two decimal places. In interpreting these it is helpful to note that for a medical school producing one hundred graduates a year, surveyed over eight years, a total of about seven hundred first career choices will be available. Averaged over the eight years, a figure of 1 per cent choices for cardiology would indicate about one graduate a year expressing this career preference.

The medical schools showing the highest average numbers of choices are: for cardiology (over 1 per cent), Cambridge, Oxford and King's College Hospital; dermatology (over 1 per cent), Sheffield and Southampton; endocrinology (0.9 per cent), the Middlesex Hospital and University College Hospital; geriatrics (over 1 per cent), Newcastle; haematology (over 2 per cent), Glasgow; nephrology (over 0.4 per cent), Middlesex Hospital and Oxford; neurology (over 1 per cent), Charing Cross Hospital, Royal Free Hospital, Oxford, University College Hospital, King's College Hospital and Cambridge; rheumatology (over 0.6 per cent), King's College Hospital, Middlesex Hospital and St Bartholomew's Hospital; thoracic medicine (over 0.8 per cent), St George's Hospital and St Mary's Hospital. For all of these medical specialties together, the highest average proportions of choices came from Cambridge, Oxford and University College Hospital; the lowest were from Belfast, Birmingham, Leicester and Aberdeen. This variation may be an indication of the extent to which students have contact with the medical specialties during their undergraduate course. The ranges within these small numbers of preferences are quite considerable; it is interesting, for example, that the average number of choices for geriatrics was twice as high in Newcastle as from any other medical school, with the exception of Bristol which came up to about three-quarters of the Newcastle level. A number of medical schools

Table 3.8 First choices of career at the pre-registration stage for surgical specialties: percentages of respondents from all years surveyed

Medical school	*Accident & emergency*	*ENT*	*Neuro-surgery*	*Ophthal-mology*	*Orthopaedics*	*Paediatric surgery*	*Plastic surgery*	*Thoracic surgery*	*Urology*	*All specialties shown*
Aberdeen	1.20	0.00	0.58	0.29	0.77	0.14	0.58	0.14	0.00	3.70
Dundee	0.49	1.33	0.30	1.43	3.37	0.22	0.64	0.00	0.30	8.08
Edinburgh	0.34	0.20	0.31	1.35	1.73	0.31	0.34	0.10	0.10	4.78
Glasgow	0.69	0.15	0.25	0.59	1.66	0.21	0.38	0.38	0.08	4.39
Birmingham	0.20	0.51	0.30	1.19	1.35	0.20	0.30	0.20	0.13	4.38
Bristol	0.92	0.10	0.06	2.08	0.87	0.31	0.18	0.04	0.06	4.62
Cambridge	0.85	0.85	0.43	3.11	3.53	0.43	0.43	1.28	0.00	10.91
Leeds	1.14	0.95	0.52	1.17	1.75	0.32	0.45	0.00	0.13	6.43
Leicester	0.00	0.86	0.00	2.59	0.43	0.00	0.00	0.00	0.00	3.88
Liverpool	0.89	0.11	0.34	1.43	2.61	0.61	0.49	0.15	0.11	6.74
Manchester	0.29	0.05	0.57	0.98	1.63	0.16	0.53	0.36	0.00	4.57
Newcastle	0.45	0.32	0.26	1.95	1.56	0.00	0.91	0.00	0.00	5.45
Nottingham	0.14	0.14	0.29	0.86	2.51	0.43	0.09	0.37	0.00	4.83
Oxford	0.47	1.76	0.23	1.83	2.72	0.23	0.89	0.47	0.23	8.83
Sheffield	0.35	0.56	0.42	1.39	2.36	0.14	0.28	0.00	0.00	5.50
Southampton	0.47	0.47	0.23	3.22	1.17	0.23	0.58	0.00	0.23	6.60

Table 3.8 continued

Medical school	*Accident & emergency*	*ENT*	*Neuro-surgery*	*Ophthal-mology*	*Orthopaedics*	*Paediatric surgery*	*Plastic surgery*	*Thoracic surgery*	*Urology*	*All specialties shown*
Charing Cross	0.56	0.75	0.19	0.84	2.36	0.00	0.56	0.09	0.19	5.54
Guy's	0.38	1.01	0.38	1.64	1.47	0.00	0.76	0.44	0.00	6.08
King's College	0.65	0.73	0.00	1.26	2.71	0.00	0.58	0.40	0.00	6.33
The London	0.69	0.51	0.27	0.88	2.52	0.34	0.72	0.23	0.14	6.30
Middlesex	0.18	0.83	0.14	1.63	2.42	0.41	0.83	0.41	0.28	7.13
Royal Free	0.64	0.48	0.16	1.33	2.01	0.00	0.56	0.32	0.16	5.66
St Bart's	0.37	0.98	0.12	1.35	2.18	0.00	0.68	0.34	0.18	6.20
St George's	0.44	0.49	0.12	1.73	1.63	0.25	0.25	0.25	0.00	5.16
St Mary's	0.15	0.61	0.31	1.11	3.39	0.00	0.53	0.31	0.15	6.56
St Thomas'	0.17	1.33	0.08	2.49	3.37	0.08	0.50	0.25	0.00	8.27
UCH	0.07	1.37	0.54	0.93	1.71	0.00	0.29	0.14	0.43	5.48
Westminster	1.52	0.62	0.00	1.51	4.35	0.27	0.41	0.41	0.00	0.09
Wales	0.57	0.57	0.38	0.88	1.70	0.13	0.19	0.25	0.00	4.67
Belfast	0.17	0.79	0.39	0.79	0.50	0.00	0.00	0.20	0.00	2.84

showed no first choices at all, over the whole eight years, for some of these medical specialties. Again, it should be remembered that the figures for Leicester relate to only two years (a total of 116 respondents).

In Table 3.7 haematology is shown among the medical specialties. This column includes all choices given as 'haematology' or as 'clinical haematology'.

Table 3.8 deals with the surgical specialties in a similar way. Once again, the ranges are very considerable with the average percentages of first choices for all the surgical specialties shown varying from almost eleven from Cambridge and over nine from Westminster Hospital to fewer than four from Leicester, Aberdeen and Belfast. Belfast and Aberdeen are the medical schools which notably produced fewer career choices for either surgical or medical specialties.

Among individual surgical specialties the highest average percentages of choices for accident and emergency came from Westminster Hospital, Aberdeen and Leeds, with the lowest from University College Hospital and, perhaps interestingly in relation to the prevalence of civil disturbance, Belfast. The highest proportions of choices for ENT surgery (over 1 per cent) came from Oxford, University College Hospital, St Thomas' Hospital, Dundee and Guy's Hospital. Neurosurgery featured relatively prominently among qualifiers from Aberdeen, Manchester, Leeds and University College Hospital. Ophthalmology attracted an average of more than 3 per cent of first choices among qualifiers from Southampton and Cambridge, and only 0.29 per cent from Aberdeen. There was an average of over 4 per cent first choices for orthopaedics from Westminster Hospital, and over 3 per cent from Dundee, Cambridge, St Mary's Hospital and St Thomas' Hospital. From Belfast, Bristol and Aberdeen the figure was less than 1 per cent. Liverpool produced the highest average proportion of choices for paediatric surgery, and Cambridge outstandingly the highest proportion for cardiothoracic surgery. Interest in plastic surgery was perhaps surprisingly high and evenly distributed in relation to some of the specialties which might have been expected to be more familiar to students. Interest in urology was very limited, the highest average figure, from University College Hospital, being less than 0.5 per cent.

CHANGES OF CAREER CHOICE

Tables 3.9 to 3.12 relate to 1974 and 1977 qualifiers. They give a general picture of how often changes of career choices occurred and at what stages after graduation. Therefore, data are included only for doctors who responded to every two-yearly questionnaire. In these tables all changes of specialty or mainstream are shown as whole changes of choice even where ties of choice were involved, for example medicine tied with general practice as a first choice in 1975, followed by a straight first choice for general practice in 1977 would be counted as a change of mainstream in Table 3.9 and as a change of specialty in Table 3.10. Allowing for this, and also for the fact that indefinite choices are included, these tables may be said to maximize the number of 'changes of choice' that were reported.

The end columns of the tables show the cumulative percentages of doctors who had signified by their replies various numbers of changes of first choice (including returns to a previous choice). The 1977 qualifiers, followed for seven years, show a slightly higher percentage with no changes of choice than the 1974 qualifiers who were followed for eleven years. These extra four years represent two additional surveys, so that the possible number of recorded changes of choice is three for the 1977 cohort and five for the 1974 cohort. The vertical lines in the tables show the percentages of these respondents who made a change of choice between consecutive surveys. The commonest time for changes to occur was within the first three years of qualifying. The tables for 1974 qualifiers (Tables 3.9 and 3.10) show that changes of choice became comparatively infrequent after seven years.

Tables 3.9 and 3.11 show changes of choice by mainstream and Tables 3.10 and 3.12 show changes by specific specialty. About half the original choices of these doctors remained within the same *mainstream* after seven years; about a third made one change of mainstream and fewer than 5 per cent made more than two such changes. Only about one-third of the original choices adhered specifically to the same *specialty* after seven years; at this stage about 10 per cent of respondents had made three changes of specialty choice, that is, their choice had changed on every occasion when they had responded. After eleven years the 1974 respondents included about 20 per cent with more than two *specialty* changes; twenty respondents had changed their choice on all five surveys.

Table 3.9 Changes of mainstream choice among doctors responding to every two-year survey (1974 qualifiers: 1,006 doctors)

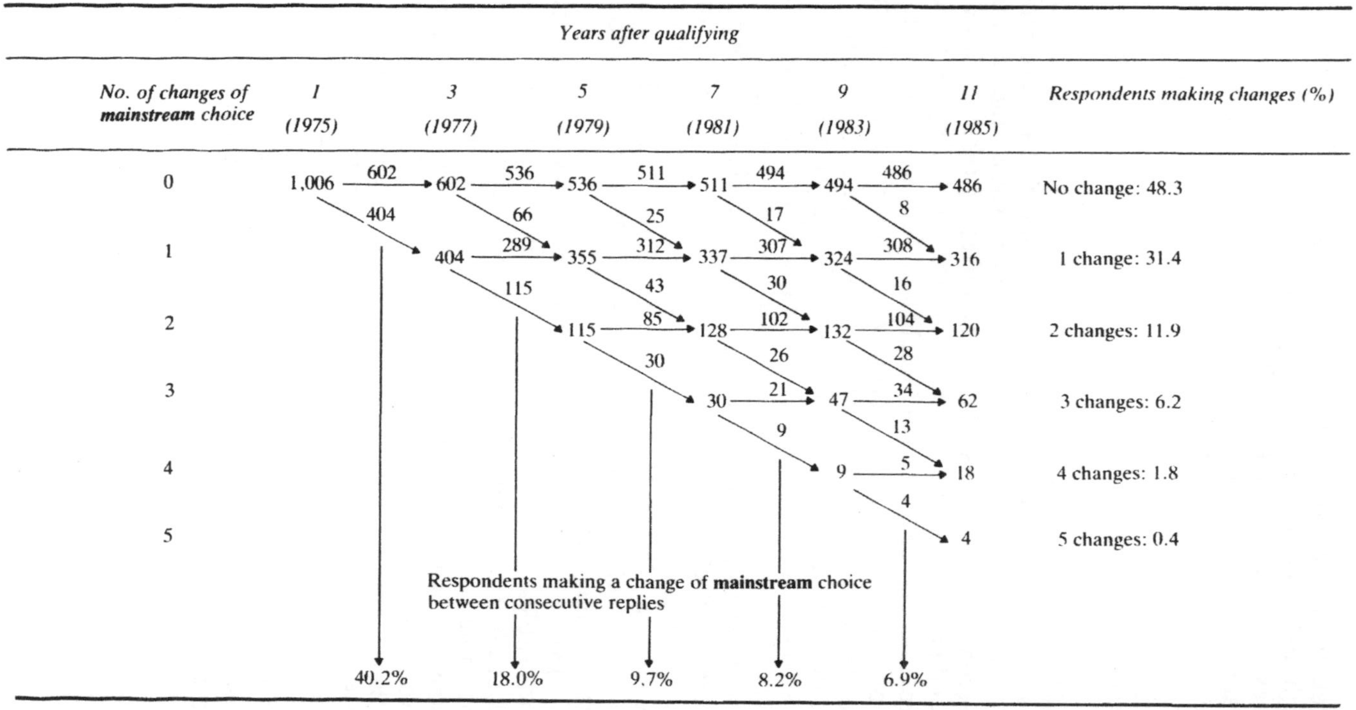

Years after qualifying
No. of changes of **mainstream** choice
1 *(1975)*
3 *(1977)*
5 *(1979)*
7 *(1981)*
9 *(1983)*
11 *(1985)*
Respondents making changes (%)
0
1,006
602
602
536
536
511
511
494
494
486
486
No change: 48.3
404
66
25
17
8
1
404
289
355
312
337
307
324
308
316
1 change: 31.4
115
43
30
16
2
115
85
128
102
132
104
120
2 changes: 11.9
30
26
28
3
30
21
47
34
62
3 changes: 6.2
9
13
4
9
5
18
4 changes: 1.8
4
5
4
5 changes: 0.4
Respondents making a change of **mainstream** choice between consecutive replies
40.2%
18.0%
9.7%
8.2%
6.9%

Table 3.10 Changes of specialty choice among doctors responding to every two-year survey (1974 qualifiers: 1,006 doctors)

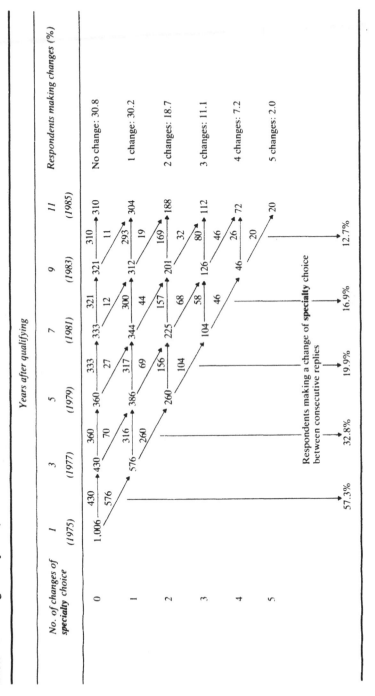

No. of changes of **specialty** *choice*	*Years after qualifying* 1 (1975)		3 (1977)		5 (1979)		7 (1981)		9 (1983)		11 (1985)	*Respondents making changes (%)*
0	1,006	430 →; 576 ↘	430	360 →; 70 ↘	360	333 →; 27 ↘	333	321 →; 12 ↘	321	310 →; 11 ↘	310	No change: 30.8
1			576	316 →; 260 ↘	386	317 →; 69 ↘	344	300 →; 44 ↘	312	293 →; 19 ↘	304	1 change: 30.2
2					260	156 →; 104 ↘	225	157 →; 68 ↘	201	169 →; 32 ↘	188	2 changes: 18.7
3							104	58 →; 46 ↘	126	80 →; 46 ↘	112	3 changes: 11.1
4									46	26 →; 20 ↘	72	4 changes: 7.2
5											20	5 changes: 2.0
Respondents making a change of **specialty** choice between consecutive replies		57.3%		32.8%		19.9%		16.9%		12.7%		

Table 3.11 Changes of mainstream choice among doctors responding to every two-year survey (1977 qualifiers: 1,859 doctors)

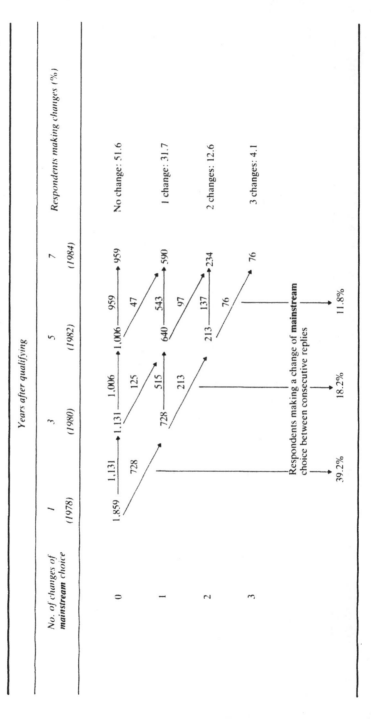

	Years after qualifying							
No. of changes of ***mainstream*** *choice*	*1* (*1978*)		*3* (*1980*)		*5* (*1982*)		*7* (*1984*)	*Respondents making changes (%)*
0	1,859	1,131 →	1,131	1,006 →	1,006	959 →	959	No change: 51.6
		728 ↘		125 ↘		47 ↘		
1			728	515 →	640	543 →	590	1 change: 31.7
				213 ↘		97 ↘		
2					213	137 →	234	2 changes: 12.6
						76 ↘		
3							76	3 changes: 4.1
Respondents making a change of **mainstream** choice between consecutive replies		39.2%		18.2%		11.8%		

Table 3.12 Changes of specialty choice among doctors responding to every two-year survey (1977 qualifiers: 1,859 doctors)

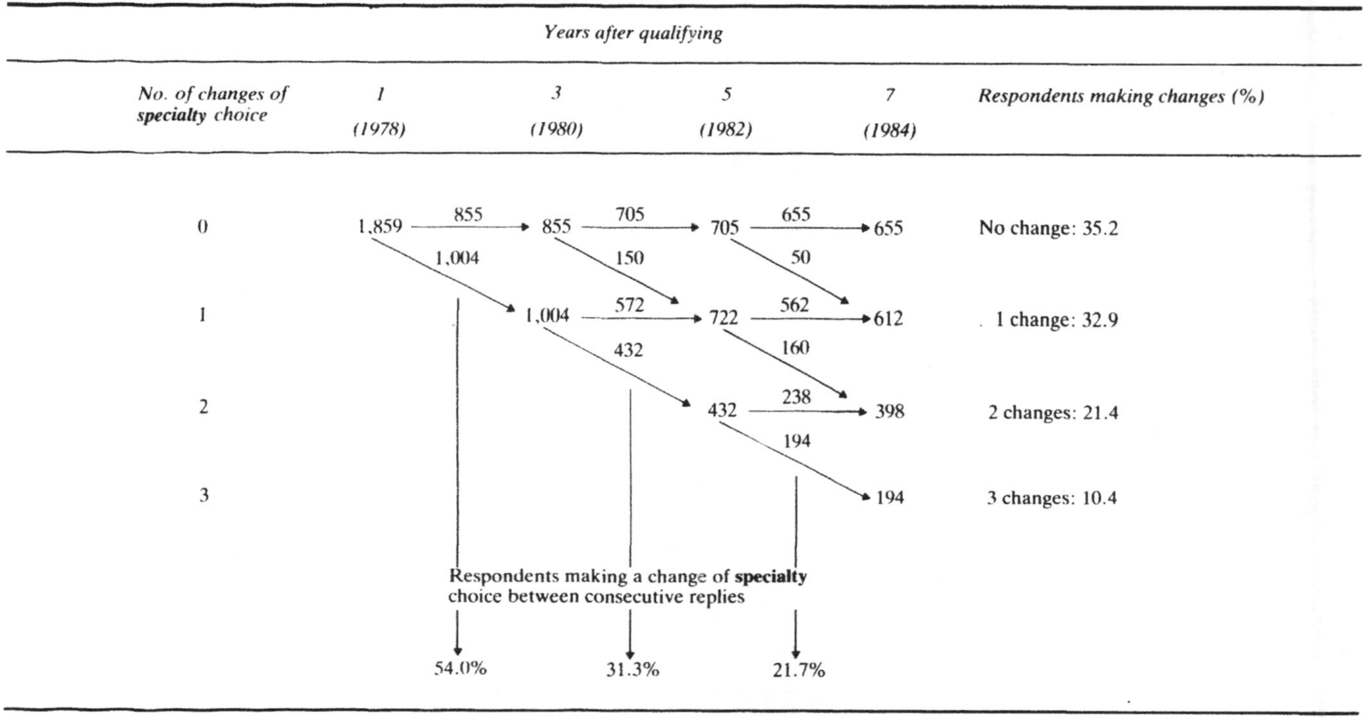

Table 3.13 First choice of career (corrected for ties): changes of mainstream between 1975 and 1981 (1974 qualifiers)

1981	*Medicine*	*Paed-iatrics*	*Surgery*	*Obstet-rics & gynae-cology*	*GP ± other*	*Psych-iatry*	*Community medicine*
1975							
Medicine	145.5	16.5	14.0	2.3	121.7	13.5	2.5
Paediatrics	7.2	37.8	1.5	1.0	48.2	1.0	9.2
Surgery	11.1	1.0	153.2	2.0	58.8		1.6
Obst. & Gynaec.	3.6	0.5	4.3	26.8	19.3	0.5	1.8
GP ± other	13.3	4.2	7.0	8.3	479.9	19.5	15.5
Psychiatry	1.0		0.3		10.5	38.5	2.5
Comm. medicine	0.3		0.5		4.2	1.0	2.2
Pathology	7.0	0.5	1.5		10.0	0.5	3.5
Anaesthetics	1.5	0.5	0.5		16.2	1.0	
Radiology	2.3			1.0	7.3		
Radiotherapy	2.0	1.0			4.8	2.0	2.0
Other medical	1.5	1.3	3.2	1.0	13.7	0.5	1.5
Non-medical	1.0				2.3		
Corrected first choices in 1981							
Number	197.3	63.3	186.0	42.5	797.0	78.0	42.2
% of all choices	11.8	3.8	11.1	2.5	47.7	4.7	2.5
% point change 1975-81	-10.2	-3.0	-4.5	-1.4	+12.3	+1.2	+2.0

Note: a Percentages calculated with a base of <50 choices corrected for ties
Source: Adapted from Parkhouse and Ellin 1988a by permission from the *BMJ*

Changes of choice by specialty group

Table 3.13 shows first choices of career of 1974 qualifiers in 1975 and in 1981 — one and seven years after qualifying (Parkhouse and Ellin 1988a). Table 3.14 shows comparable data for 1977 qualifiers, that is, in 1978 and 1984.

Data are available for individual specialties, but, to avoid formidable complexity, choices are here grouped into mainstreams. Actual changes are thus under-represented in these tables, for example a change from endocrinology to gastroenterology (both in the 'medicine' mainstream), from

Pathology	Anaes-thetics	Radio-logy	Radio-therapy	Other medical	Non-medical	Corrected first choices in 1975 Number	% of all choices	Unchanged choices in 1981 (%)
14.0	10.3	12.3	6.0	8.7	0.3	367.7	22.0	39.6
1.0	1.8	1.7	2.0	1.3		113.7	6.8	33.2
4.5	19.7	4.0	2.0	2.0	1.0	260.8	15.6	58.7
1.0	3.2	1.5		2.0		64.5	3.9	41.6
7.0	18.3	5.8	2.0	3.6	7.3	591.8	35.4	81.1
1.0	1.3		1.0	1.3	0.5	58.0	3.5	66.4
0.3					0.3	8.8	0.5	25.0[a]
32.7	1.7	1.7		1.0	1.0	61.0	3.7	53.6
0.5	45.3	1.0	1.0	1.0	1.0	69.5	4.2	65.2
	1.3	9.2		0.3		21.5	1.3	42.8[a]
0.5	0.3	0.3	1.0	0.3		14.2	0.8	7.0[a]
1.0			1.0	7.5		32.2	1.9	23.3[a]
					3.0	6.3	0.4	47.6[a]
63.5	103.3	37.5	16.0	28.8	14.5	1,670.0		
3.8	6.2	2.2	1.0	1.7	0.9		100.0	
+0.1	+2.0	+0.9	+0.2	-0.2	+0.5			

orthopaedics to ENT (both in the 'surgery' mainstream), or microbiology to chemical pathology (both in the 'pathology' mainstream) do not appear in the tables.

The margins of the tables show the gains and losses for each specialty during the period between the pre-registration year and the time when career paths began to stabilize to some extent. For example, among 1974 qualifiers 22.0 per cent of corrected first choices were for medicine in 1975 and only 11.8 per cent in 1981. The body of the tables shows where movements of choice took place: most of the losses from medicine among 1974 doctors were to general practice and, much less commonly, to a variety of specialties including paediatrics, pathology, surgery and

Table 3.14 First choice of career (corrected for ties): changes of mainstream between 1978 and 1984 (1977 qualifiers)

1984	*Medicine*	*Paed-iatrics*	*Surgery*	*Obstet-rics & gynae-cology*	*GP ± other*	*Psych-iatry*	*Community medicine*
1978							
Medicine	165.1	14.3	13.8	1.7	145.9	12.3	8.3
Paediatrics	8.8	41.3	3.0	0.7	47.9	5.5	9.5
Surgery	11.3	2.5	225.8	6.7	93.2	2.5	4.5
Obst. & gynaec.	2.0	0.8	3.0	26.7	22.5	4.5	2.0
GP ± other	16.4	4.8	8.2	6.8	635.4	24.8	20.9
Psychiatry	2.8				15.5	58.8	4.3
Comm. medicine	1.0				6.2	1.0	9.3
Pathology	6.1	0.3	1.0		13.3	1.0	4.5
Anaesthetics	4.5		2.3		31.8	1.3	5.8
Radiology	3.0		1.3		10.2		2.3
Radiotherapy	1.3	2.0		1.0	7.2		
Other medical	6.8	1.5	4.0	1.0	13.8	3.7	1.0
Non-medical	1.0				2.0	3.2	2.3
Corrected first choices in 1984							
Number	230.2	67.5	262.5	44.5	1,045.0	118.7	74.8
% of all choices	10.2	3.0	11.7	2.0	46.5	5.3	3.3
% point change 1978-84	-9.9	-2.7	-5.9	-1.1	+11.9	+1.5	+2.4

Note: a Percentages calculated with a base of <50 choices corrected for ties

psychiatry. Gains for medicine, as seen in the first column of the tables, were principally from general practice, surgery and paediatrics. The final column of the tables indicates persistence of choice — the percentage of choices for a mainstream at the pre-registration stage which remained with the same mainstream six years later.

There is great similarity between 1974 and 1977 qualifiers in the distribution of career choices, the pattern of changes and, allowing for the effect of small numbers in some mainstreams, in the degree of persistence of different choices.

						Corrected first choices in 1978		
Pathology	*Anaes-thetics*	*Radio-logy*	*Radio-therapy*	*Other medical*	*Non-medical*	*Number*	*% of all choices*	*Unchanged choices in 1984 (%)*
27.0	15.7	26.3	10.0	10.5	1.5	452.5	20.1	36.5
4.5	4.7	1.0	2.0		0.3	129.2	5.7	32.0
8.0	20.8	15.0	1.0	3.0	1.3	395.7	17.6	57.1
	2.8	1.0	1.0	3.0		69.3	3.1	38.5
6.3	25.7	8.8	2.0	12.3	5.8	778.3	34.6	81.6
2.0	0.3			2.3	0.3	86.5	3.8	68.0
		0.5	0.5	1.3		19.8	0.9	47.0[a]
46.3	1.0	1.3		2.3	0.5	77.7	3.5	59.6
1.0	66.5	1.0	0.5	4.0		118.8	5.3	56.0
0.3	2.0	15.0	0.5	1.3		36.0	1.6	41.7[a]
	1.0		5.0		0.5	18.0	0.8	27.8[a]
4.0	3.0		1.0	12.8		52.7	2.3	24.3
		1.0		3.0	2.0	14.5	0.6	13.8[a]
99.5	143.5	71.0	23.5	56.0	12.3	2249.0		
4.4	6.4	3.2	1.0	2.5	0.5		100.0	
+0.9	+1.1	+1.6	+0.2	+0.2	-0.1			

The most obvious feature in both these tables is movement towards general practice coupled with a very high persistence of initial choices for general practice (over 80 per cent). Gains for general practice were predominantly from medicine, paediatrics and surgery. Most other mainstreams showed some gain in their proportion of choices. Radiology and radiotherapy, for example, gained largely from medicine, general practice and surgery; anaesthetics attracted most new choices from surgery and general practice but also lost substantially to general practice; movement into pathology was mainly from medicine. Only about 40 per cent of initial choices for obstetrics and gynaecology, and fewer than 40 per cent of those from medicine and paediatrics, persisted after six years.

Table 3.15 Importance of various factors in years shown (1974 qualifiers)[a]

Factors	*1981*			*1983*			*1985*		
	0	*1*	*2*	*0*	*1*	*2*	*0*	*1*	*2*
Domestic circumstances	35	26	40	33	26	41	32	26	43
Financial circumstances	54	32	15	53	32	16	49	34	18
Promotion prospects/difficulties	26	38	37	22	40	39	21	38	41
Aptitude/ability	15	25	60	10	23	67	8	22	71
Advice	54	37	9	51	39	10	45	44	12
Undergraduate experience	61	25	15	58	27	16	54	28	18
Department/teacher contact	58	23	19	54	24	22	50	26	24
Pre-medical school inclinations	69	16	15	66	20	14	65	20	15
Experience of previous choice	57	22	21	54	25	21	59	24	17
Experience of present choice	42	18	40	43	18	39	21	20	59
Other reasons	83	6	11	84	6	10	89	2	9

Notes: a Figures are percentages of respondents with valid replies, men and women combined

0 = factor considered not important or column left blank

1 = factor considered of minor importance or column ticked

2 = factor considered of major importance

REASONS FOR CHOICE AND CHANGE OF CHOICE

When we wrote in 1979 to the doctors who qualified in 1974 we asked respondents who had changed their choice of career since the pre-registration year to indicate, from a list, one or more reasons which had influenced them (Parkhouse *et al.* 1981a). Of all those who replied (75 per cent of the identified 1974 qualifiers), 41.4 per cent gave reasons for a change of first choice of career. Postgraduate experience, awareness of promotion prospects and problems, and self-appraisal appeared as the most common factors, with altered domestic circumstances featuring somewhat less prominently and careers advice or altered financial circumstances having comparatively little influence. For each broad specialty group, we were able to analyse gains and losses of potential recruits, as judged by shifts in career choice, showing the numbers of people influenced in each case by the various listed factors.

Table 3.16 Importance of various factors in years shown (1977 qualifiers)[a]

Factors	*1982*			*1984*		
	0	*1*	*2*	*0*	*1*	*2*
Domestic circumstances	35	27	39	31	28	41
Financial circumstances	55	34	11	55	32	13
Promotion prospects/difficulties	17	37	46	18	38	44
Aptitude/ability	9	22	68	8	20	72
Advice	45	44	11	44	45	11
Undergraduate experience	51	30	19	54	30	17
Department/teacher contact	54	25	20	54	27	19
Pre-medical school inclinations	67	19	14	67	20	13
Experience of previous choice	54	22	23	54	25	20
Experience of present choice	38	20	42	19	22	59
Other reasons	83	6	11	89	3	8

Notes: a Figures are percentages of respondents with valid replies, men and women combined
0 = factor considered not important or column left blank
1 = factor considered of minor importance or column ticked
2 = factor considered of major importance

From 1979 onwards we included in our surveys questions about factors which had influenced choice of career, regardless of whether any changes of career preference had occurred, thus giving all our respondents a chance to comment. The relevant item in these later questionnaires is shown in the example (Appendix, pp. 315-16).

For each possible reason, respondents were asked to indicate, 0 = Not important; 1 = Minor importance; 2 = Major importance.

If a box was left blank this was taken to signify 0 (not important) and if a box was ticked this was regarded as equivalent to 1 (minor importance). The numbers of blanks, ticks and spoiled entries was in fact very low in all cases, except that for 'other' reasons the relevant box was often left blank.

Table 3.15 gives a picture of the degree of importance assigned to various reasons for choice or change of choice by 1974 qualifiers, seven, nine and eleven years after graduation. Table 3.16 gives the same picture for 1977 qualifiers five and seven years after graduation. The similarities between 1974 and

Table 3.17 Male 1974 qualifiers in 1981 (1,396 doctors with valid career choices)[a]

Factors	*Medicine*	*Paediat-rics* [b]	*Surgery*	*Obstet. & Gynaecol.*[b]	*GP ± other*
Domestic circumstances	20	22	15	21	46
Financial circumstances	4	5	7	3	29
Promotion prospects/difficulties	41	18	27	33	44
Aptitude/ability	61	54	68	43	59
Advice	22	19	23	11	5
Undergraduate experience	14	32	23	41	8
Department/teacher contact	44	45	33	27	7
Pre-medical school inclinations	3	6	18	6	23
Experience of previous choice	24	24	20	13	20
Experience of present choice	47	47	46	29	38
Other reasons	13	16	11	6	9

Notes: a Numbers indicate percentages of respondents with valid career choices who considered given factors to be of *major importance*; allocation of reasons to mainstreams allows for tied choices of career

b Percentages based on <50 choices corrected for ties

c Percentages based on <25 choices corrected for ties

Table 3.18 Female 1974 qualifiers in 1981 (540 doctors with valid career choices)[a]

Factors	*Medicine*[b]	*Paediat-rics*[b]	*Surgery*[c]	*Obstet. & Gynaecol.*[c]	*GP ± other*
Domestic circumstances	52	40	42	12	71
Financial circumstances	4	0	6	0	10
Promotion prospects/difficulties	35	4	23	4	37
Aptitude/ability	58	53	71	60	60
Advice	2	6	17	16	4
Undergraduate experience	18	29	23	40	11
Department/teacher contact	37	28	31	44	7
Pre-medical school inclinations	0	0	12	24	14
Experience of previous choice	24	20	35	16	21
Experience of present choice	35	32	35	40	36
Other reasons	12	12	0	16	10

Notes: a Numbers indicate percentages of respondents with valid career choices who considered given factors to be of *major importance*; allocation of reasons to mainstreams allows for tied choices of career

b Percentages based on <50 choices corrected for ties

c Percentages based on <25 choices corrected for ties

Psych- iatry	Comm. med.[c]	Pathology	Anaes- thetics	Radio- logy[b]	Radio- therapy[c]	Other medical[b]	Non- medical[c]
12	33	27	17	33	18	35	47
5	6	7	7	2	0	35	55
22	33	40	38	54	35	51	47
77	66	65	71	53	47	66	62
0	16	16	10	13	6	11	0
33	0	16	25	0	6	14	12
29	22	33	26	13	35	6	3
33	22	9	1	0	0	28	16
21	40	16	22	33	29	34	47
39	22	48	51	46	41	51	26
10	35	11	9	10	6	29	34

Psych- iatry[b]	Comm. med.[b]	Pathology[c]	Anaes- thetics[b]	Radio- logy[c]	Radio- therapy[c]	Other medical[c]	Non- medical[c]
32	86	42	36	38	33	27	60
3	3	4	11	0	0	13	0
19	26	36	39	56	44	47	0
68	49	67	64	31	67	73	60
4	2	9	4	6	0	13	0
33	14	36	18	0	11	0	40
17	18	27	11	31	44	27	0
11	13	9	0	0	0	0	40
28	25	22	14	6	33	47	20
49	33	40	43	44	56	27	40
15	9	9	18	13	0	33	20

Table 3.19 Male 1977 qualifiers in 1984 (1,657 doctors with valid career choices)[a]

Factors	*Medicine*	*Paediatrics*[b]	*Surgery*	*Obstet. & Gynaecol.*[b]	*GP ± other*
Domestic circumstances	22	8	17	8	51
Financial circumstances	7	3	6	8	27
Promotion prospects/difficulties	39	21	31	19	53
Aptitude/ability	68	77	77	89	68
Advice	18	23	23	14	6
Undergraduate experience	20	18	26	54	12
Department/teacher contact	43	41	32	51	6
Pre-medical school inclinations	5	3	13	5	19
Experience of previous choice	16	13	16	11	20
Experience of present choice	61	74	68	76	50
Other reasons	13	10	4	8	7

Notes: a Numbers indicate percentages of respondents with valid career choices who considered given factors to be of *major importance*; allocation of reasons to mainstreams allows for tied choices of career

b Percentages based on <50 choices corrected for ties

c Percentages based on <25 choices corrected for ties

Table 3.20 Female 1977 qualifiers in 1984 (856 doctors with valid career choices)[a]

Factors	*Medicine*	*Paediatrics*[b]	*Surgery*[b]	*Obstet. & Gynaecol.*[c]	*GP ± other*
Domestic circumstances	35	25	38	28	65
Financial circumstances	3	0	0	5	8
Promotion prospects/difficulties	42	19	40	13	43
Aptitude/ability	66	68	78	68	75
Advice	28	13	16	20	7
Undergraduate experience	18	23	29	33	11
Department/teacher contact	33	27	44	20	6
Pre-medical school inclinations	2	14	0	0	16
Experience of previous choice	23	4	13	20	23
Experience of present choice	66	72	71	73	60
Other reasons	1	4	13	0	5

Notes: a Numbers indicate percentages of respondents with valid career choices who considered given factors to be of *major importance*; allocation of reasons to mainstreams allows for tied choices of career

b Percentages based on <50 choices corrected for ties

c Percentages based on <25 choices corrected for ties

Psychiatry	*Comm. med.*[c]	*Pathology*	*Anaesthetics*	*Radiology*	*Radiotherapy*[c]	*Other medical*[b]	*Non-medical*[c]
15	44	34	14	32	11	35	63
3	4	6	7	9	0	21	38
36	51	61	48	88	60	51	25
85	74	77	88	50	68	71	50
8	9	10	9	13	22	25	0
35	4	18	21	9	16	22	0
36	9	32	27	18	35	20	0
28	17	9	6	2	5	18	0
23	34	18	19	18	5	41	38
64	49	53	63	38	65	62	50
12	19	9	9	7	11	29	63

Psychiatry	*Comm. med.*	*Pathology*[b]	*Anaesthetics*	*Radiology*[c]	*Radiotherapy*[c]	*Other medical*[c]	*Non-medical*[c]
47	69	37	36	38	32	54	25
7	13	1	5	0	0	17	19
39	35	40	41	63	32	32	19
91	65	67	73	54	81	71	63
15	5	6	12	17	3	9	19
26	3	19	12	13	13	12	0
32	9	27	29	29	10	9	0
21	13	13	0	0	10	9	0
32	33	14	14	17	29	43	56
66	56	57	66	50	77	69	56
4	14	7	7	4	19	32	38

1977 responses are striking, as also is the fact that the absolute and relative importance of various factors remained constant during the period of five to eleven years after qualifying. The only exception, as might reasonably be expected, was that experience of the current choice of career tended to become an increasingly important factor as the years passed.

Tables 3.17 to 3.20 concentrate on replies seven years after graduation in order to give a more detailed analysis of reasons, for men and women qualifiers of 1974 and 1977 separately, by mainstream. For this analysis respondents were considered to belong to the mainstream of their first choice at the time of the seven-year reply, but where there were ties of choice involving more than one mainstream, reasons were appropriately apportioned between the mainstreams concerned. Only reasons rated as of major importance are included (Parkhouse and Ellin 1988a).

Domestic circumstances assume their greatest importance as a factor among those choosing general practice and community medicine. Financial circumstances were not generally regarded as of great importance except in general practice and, interestingly, in the various 'other' medical and non-medical career choices. Promotion prospects were poorly rated as a factor in paediatrics and, among women, in obstetrics and gynaecology; but there were fewer large differences between specialties than might be expected. Self-evaluation of aptitudes and ability were clearly a major factor throughout, and emerged most highly in psychiatry. Advice from others was generally accorded little importance. Undergraduate experience was a notably relevant factor in obstetrics and gynaecology and also in psychiatry. Any dominant influence which undergraduate contact with the 'major' disciplines of medicine and surgery may have had did not appear to have persisted seven years after leaving medical school. The very low level of importance of undergraduate experience, or of contact with a specific department or individual in the choice of general practice as a career is notable among these graduates of the mid-1970s. Inclinations before entering medical school were rated most commonly as being important in psychiatry and general practice; in obstetrics and gynaecology and paediatrics the influence of this factor among women varied in the two cohorts, but the numbers of female respondents with these choices were fairly small. Experience of a previous career choice had had its greatest influence among those choosing community medicine, and 'other' medical or non-medical careers where 'other reasons' for the choice were also prominent.

It is interesting to relate these findings to the importance attributed to various factors in the self-evaluation studies reported in Chapter 15.

More recent qualifiers

At the time when our 1974 and 1977 respondents were reporting on their career choices seven years after qualifying, the graduates of 1980 and 1983 were at the pre-registration stage. Table 3.21 shows the rating of importance given by these doctors to various factors influencing their first career choices immediately after leaving medical school. Perceived aptitude and ability was the factor most commonly regarded as very important, and there appeared to be about as much regard for promotion prospects and difficulties as among more senior doctors in the early 1980s; however, the importance of undergraduate experience in determining career choice was very much stronger than after the intervention of several years of postgraduate medical practice.

Table 3.21 Importance of various factors at the pre-registration stage (1980 and 1983 qualifiers)[a]

Factors	*1980 qualifiers in 1983*			*1983 qualifiers in 1984*		
	0	*1*	*2*	*0*	*1*	*2*
Domestic circumstances	49	28	24	46	27	27
Financial circumstances	69	27	4	67	28	6
Promotion prospects/difficulties	17	39	44	14	37	49
Aptitude/ability	8	26	67	8	22	70
Advice	31	52	17	28	54	19
Undergraduate experience	24	35	41	20	35	45
Department/teacher contact	45	34	21	47	33	20
Pre-medical school inclinations	60	23	18	58	23	19
Other reasons	88	3	9	89	3	7

Notes: a Figures are percentages of respondents with valid replies, men and women combined
0 = factor considered not important or column left blank
1 = factor considered of minor importance or column ticked
2 = factor considered of major importance

COMMENT

It is worth quoting again (see Parkhouse 1978) the words of the late Sir Derrick Dunlop (1975) which so broadly placed in context the intrinsic factors contributing to career choice: 'The catholic mantle of a medical qualification, provided we don it right, can be made to fit all our tastes, talents and idiosyncrasies'. Extrinsic factors also operate, and increasingly so during the early years after graduation. Throughout this chapter the term 'career choice' is used, but one must be aware of the fact that chance, or the pressure of circumstances, often play at least as large a part in the taking-up of a particular type of work as premeditated choice. Indeed, the uninhibited career choices of young doctors form a distribution which is far from matching the needs of the service and the community. Making the dreams of every medical graduate come true, if it were possible, would lead to chaos. Whether the doctors who succeed in obtaining various career jobs are the best suited candidates for them, by reason of their ability, their need for employment, or their potential long-term work contribution is an interesting and highly debatable question. A survey of our respondents in ten or twenty years' time would perhaps reveal much useful information about job satisfaction, stress, mobility, and employment among the middle-aged doctors in our society.

It is also possible that when career choice is still indefinite, as it often is at the pre-registration stage (Johnson and Elston 1978; Egerton 1979; Parkhouse *et al.* 1983a), the preferences put down by respondents may reflect the job they are doing at the time. Change of choice may be little more than a shift from one inchoate vision to another, or from one exciting and rewarding specialty to the next.

A large literature has built up in many countries on career choice among medical students and doctors. Student preferences were studied by Martin and Boddy (1962), by the Association for the Study of Medical Education and the National Foundation for Educational Research in 1966 for the Royal Commission on Medical Education (1968), and subsequently by many others (e.g. Egerton 1979). The influence of personality characteristics (e.g. Schumacher 1964) and medical students' beliefs about different specialties (Furnham 1986) are among the factors considered to influence these early and tentative choices. The determinants of career choice among qualified doctors were reviewed by Hutt (1976) and have been studied in particular samples of graduates by Last and Stanley (1968), Hutt *et al.* (1979), Johnson and Elston (1978), Egerton (1980), MacFarlene and Parry (1979) and others. Among the conclusions of Hutt *et al.* (1979), arising from personal interviews, were varying opinions of particular specialties: e.g. surgery was considered exciting and productive of good results, anaesthetics was felt to have a good career structure, paediatrics involved awareness of the huge responsibility of losing a patient. Johnson and Elston (1978) were among the authors noting sex differences: job availability and financial circumstances mattered more to their male respondents and the possibility of part-time work was important to many women respondents. Egerton (1985) also noted that her male respondents were more preoccupied than females with security and the material and physical aspects of work. Last and Stanley (1968) compared the choices of medical students at various stages of the undergraduate course with their subsequent choices after graduation, and thus obtained data on the persistence of career choice at an earlier stage of training than our present study.

Most of the detailed information in this chapter will concern readers with an interest in a particular specialty, or medical school, or a potential influencing factor in career choice. One general point which comes out strongly is the lack of influence attributed to career advice. As things stand this is hardly surprising, because much advice is haphazard, prejudiced in favour of a specific career, or frankly ill-founded. In many cases doctors have felt safer fending for themselves by all means available to them, and the importance of this is often seen as the soundest of all advice. But guiding people on the next move, or about how best to proceed generally in order to get a particular job or succeed in a given specialty is fundamentally different from counselling people about how to understand their own inner strengths and weaknesses, how to come to terms with their professional lives and give their most valuable contribution to medicine in the light of all the wide range of help that society seeks from qualified doctors. Here is the ultimate challenge of 'career choice', which involves looking hard at the way our system operates, and at the true potentialities of the people within it.

4 Career progress

Intercalated degrees

In recent years, financial constraints have bitten more and more deeply into medical education and research (R. Smith 1988; Alexander 1988). This has created concern about the fate of the intercalated degree (R. Smith 1986; Harris 1986). Critical comments have been made about the way students are chosen for intercalated degree courses, the research content of the courses, and the reporting of outcomes (R. Smith 1986). For these reasons medical schools have been challenged to justify their claims for funding to continue the intercalated degree programme, and attempts have been made to assess the value of these degrees (Wyllie and Currie 1986; Eaton and Thong 1985; Wakeford *et al.* 1985; Evered *et al.* 1987).

We looked at our 1974 and 1977 qualifiers (Parkhouse and Ellin 1988b). We excluded students who took the pre-clinical part of the course at St Andrew's, and also Nottingham students, since in both cases a BSc was taken as a standard part of the course rather than an option. We also excluded Edinburgh qualifiers because our data did not always enable us to distinguish those who took a general BSc as a standard part of the course from those who intercalated an optional honours BSc. In fact, a study of the Edinburgh honours BSc in pathology has been published by Wyllie and Currie (1986). We treated Oxford and Cambridge pre-clinical students as a separate group, and divided the remainder of the qualifiers, from all medical schools except the ones excluded as above, into those with and without an optional intercalated degree.

THE STARTING-POINT

Table 4.1 shows that for 1974 qualifiers 15.9 per cent of men and 14.0 per cent of women took optional intercalated degrees; in 1977 the proportion of women (8.6 per cent) showed a greater decline than that of men (13.1 per cent). Overall, we identified

Table 4.1 Numbers of qualifiers showing Oxbridge graduates and those with optional intercalated degrees

Year of qualifying		*No intercalated degree*[a]	*Optional intercalated degree*[a]	*Oxbridge*	*Uncertain*	*Total*[b]
1974	Men	995	205 (15.9%)	231	93	1,524
	Women	435	74 (14.0%)	44	18	571
	Total	1,430	279 (15.3%)	275	111	2,095
1977	Men	1,298	210 (13.1%)	252	93	1,853
	Women	729	72 (8.6%)	58	35	894
	Total	2,027	282 (11.6%)	310	128	2,747

Notes: a With percentage of total minus Oxbridge graduates
b Excluding qualifiers from Edinburgh, Nottingham and St Andrew's

Table 4.2 Percentages of qualifiers (excluding Oxbridge graduates) with optional intercalated degrees, by location of medical school

Year of qualifying	*London medical schools*	*English provincial medical schools*	*Scottish medical schools*	*University of Wales College of Medicine*	*Queen's University, Belfast*
1974	22.8	11.0	7.8	11.5	
1977	20.9	7.4	6.3	0.9	5.3
1974 and 1977 combined	21.8	8.9	6.9	5.4	

15.3 per cent of qualifiers from the medical schools included in the study who had taken optional intercalated degrees and qualified in 1974, and 11.6 per cent who did so in 1977.

Table 4.3 First choices of career at pre-registration stage (corrected for ties) as percentages of all first choices of career

Specialty	*No intercalated degree*			*Optional intercalated degree*			*Oxbridge*		
	men	*women*	*total*	*men*	*women*	*total*	*men*	*women*	*total*
Medicine and medical specialties	19.4	17.6	18.8	35.1	29.9	33.7	33.8	23.2	32.0
Paediatrics	4.7	9.0	6.2	6.1	11.0	7.4	4.1	8.6	4.9
Surgery and surgical specialties	22.3	5.1	16.5	17.9	5.9	14.7	18.2	7.9	16.4
Obstetrics and gynaecology	2.9	4.4	3.4	1.8	2.1	1.8	3.8	2.1	3.5
Other hospital specialties	11.1	16.3	12.9	15.0	15.4	15.1	9.5	18.0	11.0
General practice	34.6	42.6	37.3	17.8	23.9	19.4	23.4	33.3	25.1
Academic	0.9	0.2	0.6	3.3	6.0	4.1	3.2	1.5	2.9
Other choices	4.1	4.7	4.3	3.0	5.8	3.7	4.1	5.4	4.3

Table 4.2 shows that, when Oxford and Cambridge pre-clinical students are excluded, a much higher proportion of students from the London medical schools (21.8 per cent) took optional intercalated degrees than from the English provincial medical schools (8.9 per cent), Scottish medical schools (6.9 per cent), Wales (5.4 per cent), or Belfast (5.3 per cent for 1977). The range between individual medical schools was large: in London, from 9 per cent (1977) and 12 per cent (1974) at Charing Cross Hospital, and 10 per cent (1977) at the Royal Free to 43 per cent (1974) and 45 per cent (1977) at University College Hospital. In the English provinces the range was from nil (1977) in Liverpool and 3 per cent (1974) in Sheffield to 17 per cent (1977) and 20 per cent (1974) in Leeds. There was comparatively little variation within Scotland, Dundee showing somewhat lower percentages than Glasgow and Aberdeen. No medical school in either year was within 12 per cent of University College Hospital.

Table 4.3 shows career choices at the pre-registration stage. There was a large preponderance of choices for medicine and the medical specialties among Oxbridge graduates (32.0 per cent) and qualifiers with optional intercalated degrees (33.7 per cent) compared to other qualifiers (18.8 per cent), with no disproportionate sex differences. Men overwhelmingly outnumbered women in choices for surgery and the surgical specialties, in all three groups, and paediatrics was a more popular choice throughout among women. 'Academic' choices of career are ill-defined, but were most often indicated in some way by Oxbridge students and those with optional intercalated degrees. The other striking difference is that general practice was given as a first choice of career by 37.3 per cent of qualifiers with no optional intercalated degree, compared to 25.1 per cent of Oxbridge graduates and 19.4 per cent of qualifiers with optional intercalated degrees. In all three groups general practice was favoured more by women than by men.

CAREER PROGRESS

Tables 4.4 and 4.5 are based on the 1974 qualifiers who replied to us in 1987 and the 1977 qualifiers who replied to us in 1986.

Table 4.4 shows that while much of the specialty bias shown at the pre-registration stage (Table 4.3) is retained, career aspirations were on the whole considerably toned down with time and experience. Fewer doctors were working in medicine and the medical specialties than had initially hoped to do so, but

Table 4.4 Posts held by 1,680 1974 qualifiers in 1987 and by 2,336 1977 qualifiers in 1986 (percentage distribution between specialties for each column shown)

Specialty	*No intercalated degree*	*Optional intercalated degree*	*Oxbridge*
Medicine and medical specialties	7.4	19.4	19.3
Paediatrics	1.8	3.2	2.6
Surgery and surgical specialties	8.1	8.0	9.8
Obstetrics and gynaecology	1.6	1.2	2.4
Other hospital specialties	15.6	16.0	13.3
General practice	44.3	31.1	32.7
Academic (no specialty stated)	1.7	4.2	2.8
Abroad	8.8	7.8	9.0
Other/none	10.7	9.0	8.2

Table 4.5 Posts held by 1,680 1974 qualifiers in 1987 and by 2,336 1977 qualifiers in 1986 (percentage distribution between types of post for each row shown)

Respondents	*SHO/ registrar*	*Senior registrar*	*Consultant*	*GP principal*	*Acad- emic*	*Other/ unknown*
No intercalated degree	5.3	11.3	12.6	32.2	5.3	33.2
Optional inter- calated degree	4.2	14.0	20.8	23.4	12.6	24.8
Oxbridge	6.2	15.9	13.3	23.7	13.1	27.7

compared to those with no intercalated degrees (7.4 per cent) there were proportionately many more Oxbridge graduates (19.3 per cent) and qualifiers with optional intercalated degrees (19.4 per cent). Academic work, with no specialty indicated, was also more common among the latter two groups. Many more qualifiers without intercalated degrees were working in general practice — 44.3 per cent — compared to 32.7 per cent from Oxbridge and 31.1 per cent of those with optional intercalated degrees. The percentages of people abroad were comparable in the three groups, with no suggestion of any disproportionate loss of holders of optional intercalated degrees through emigration.

By the times of their latest replies to us in 1986 and 1987, the 1974 qualifiers had naturally progressed further than the 1977 qualifiers in the hospital-based specialties. Of 1977 qualifiers who responded 8.0 per cent were SHOs or registrars, compared to 1.5 per cent of 1974 qualifiers; 8.0 per cent of respondents from 1977 were consultants compared to 21.6 per cent from 1974. In general practice, the proportions of 1974 and 1977 qualifiers who had become principals were similar. Combining the respondents from the two years, a considerably higher proportion of those with optional intercalated degrees (20.8 per cent) had become consultants than of Oxbridge graduates (13.3 per cent) or other qualifiers (12.6 per cent). Proportionately, more than twice as many Oxbridge graduates and optional intercalated degree holders than other qualifiers were in academic posts of various kinds (Table 4.5).

POSTGRADUATE QUALIFICATIONS

Altogether, about 85 per cent of 1974 and 1977 respondents were known to have at least one postgraduate qualification of some kind (Table 4.6). Of those with optional intercalated degrees 37.4 per cent were known to hold the MRCP, and 34.7 per cent of Oxbridge graduates, compared to 14.6 per cent of other qualifiers from the two years. MD, PhD and MRC Path were more commonly held by the Oxbridge and optional intercalated degree groups than by others. The reverse was true for the MRCGP. Apart from the FRCS, there were few notable sex differences except for the MRC Path, which, among holders of optional intercalated degrees, was held by 7.8 per cent of men and no women qualifying in 1974, and by 7.1 per cent of men and 2.8 per cent of women qualifying in 1977.

Two or more of the main qualifications listed separately in Table 4.6 were held by 19 per cent of Oxbridge graduates and 16 per cent of the optional intercalated degree group, compared to 7 per cent of other qualifiers. The commonest combination among 1974 qualifiers was MD MRCP. Among 1977 Oxbridge graduates and qualifiers with no intercalated degree, the commonest combination was MRCP MRCGP; among those with optional intercalated degrees it was MD MRCP.

Table 4.6 Numbers of postgraduate qualifications per 100 respondents (1974 and 1977 qualifiers combined)

Respondents	*MRCP*	*FRCS*	*MRCOG*	*FFARCS*	*FRCR*	*MRC Path*	*MRC Psych*
No intercalated degree	14.6	10.3	2.2	6.2	2.8	2.0	4.1
Optional intercalated degree	37.4	9.1	1.1	5.2	3.0	5.9	4.6
Oxbridge	34.7	12.3	2.6	3.1	2.4	3.8	3.2
All respondents	19.9	10.4	2.1	5.7	2.8	2.7	4.1

Respondents	*MRGCP*	*MD*	*PhD/ DPhil*	*MS/ MChir*	*All other qualifications*	*None*	*Not known*	*Total no. of respondents*
No intercalated degree	20.3	2.5	0.3	0.5	109.3	11.5	6.9	3,457
Optional intercalated degree	15.7	7.3	1.8	0.4	130.5	5.0	2.9	561
Oxbridge	18.6	8.0	1.9	1.0	123.6	4.1	7.0	585
All respondents	19.5	3.8	0.7	0.6	113.7	9.8	6.5	4,603

LOCATION OF WORK

Among 1974 and 1977 qualifiers combined, 18.2 per cent of respondents in the group with no intercalated degree were working in the city of their medical school at the time of their latest reply. This contrasted with 22.7 per cent of the Oxbridge graduates (chi-square, $p<0.05$) and 25.3 per cent of the qualifiers with optional intercalated degrees ($p<0.001$). There was no appreciable difference between the three groups in regard to the percentage of non-London qualifiers who were working in Greater London (4.0, 4.4 and 4.0 per cent) or in the percentages who were not working (1.6, 1.8 and 2.3 per cent).

MARRIAGE AND CHILDREN

In 1986–87, 87.6 per cent of male respondents and 76.0 per cent of female respondents from the two years of qualifiers were married (chi-square $p<0.001$). There was no significant difference between the Oxbridge, optional intercalated degree and other groups, for men or women, in the frequency of marriage. For all respondents 19.7 per cent of men and 29.8 per cent of women did not have children; 24.3 per cent of the men and 17.1 per cent of the women had three or more children. These differences between men and women were significant ($p<0.001$) and occurred in all three groups of qualifiers, but there were no significant differences between the groups themselves.

DISCUSSION

The literature on optional intercalated degrees is full of opinions but comparatively short of facts. Richard Smith (1986) described the intercalated year as the time when people learn to think and to question and to find out things for themselves. No one, according to Smith, 'seems to dispute the value of these degrees'. Similarly Harris (1986) made the bold statement that students' 'basic attitudes to medicine are changed by their experience' of the intercalated degree.

Eaton and Thong (1985) reported that students in Queensland who took an intercalated BSc more often graduated MB with honours, more commonly held higher research degrees, and published more articles, books and chapters than other students. The authors recognized, however, that it was the more able and better motivated students who had the chance to take an intercalated degree. MacGowan *et al.* (1986) from Aberdeen gave data to support Wyllie and Currie's (1986) findings about the positive relationship between intercalated degrees and career choices for medicine and pathology, and research output. Wyllie and Currie's study showed favourable comparison of intercalated degree holders in pathology with students whose marks were lower, and also with a group sharing the academic excellence of the intercalated degree group but lacking their motivation. The question of how well the best and highly motivated students would have done without an intercalated degree clearly remains unanswered: as Smith (1986) wrote, 'many of these self-selected doctors might, of course, have gone into academic medicine anyway'. Two contrasting views of the situation are shown, by the robust defence of Wyllie and Currie (1986): 'even if this merely reflects the same drive that led them to choose the intercalated year in the first place our data strongly support the claim that the honours course is being taken by a worthy group of students'; and by Longmore:

> students who are inclined to go in for the science degree are likely to be those who would normally and naturally follow a more scientific course at the end of their medical studies. I do not see how it would be any loss to them to avoid having to do an extra year . . . it certainly puts them at an advantage and they seem to me to form part of an elite.
>
> (Longmore 1986)

Examining the question from the other end, Wakeford *et al.* (1985) found that 39 per cent of a sample of 262 doctors who were selected as being heavily involved in medical research had either an intercalated BSc or a BA (e.g. Oxbridge), compared to their estimate that not more than 10 per cent of all UK medical graduates had a BA or BSc degree. They reported a positive relationship between possession of an intercalated degree and an early decision to enter a research career. In a further paper Evered *et al.* (1987) surveyed 94 per cent of all the medically qualified professors and readers in UK medical faculties. Oxbridge graduates and holders of intercalated degrees were very strongly represented. Compared to Oxbridge and other graduates in these senior academic posts, holders of intercalated degrees raised more clinical research grants, had a better publication record and were more frequently cited. Oxbridge graduates raised the most grants in non-clinical specialties. This study provides the best control, in that it compared senior academics of identical status and different undergraduate backgrounds. The authors saw it as refuting the National Audit Office's criticism that the MRC's awards for intercalated degrees had become of 'a general educational (rather than research) nature'; they felt their study gave 'strong evidence that the intercalated BSc is of real importance in developing a cadre of trained research workers for the future'. Two points may be made: first, that research achievement is not necessarily the main criterion, and it is certainly not the only one, by which the stature of all senior academics should be judged; second, that if the intercalated BSc did not exist there would still be very able, highly motivated doctors with a major interest in research. But at least it seems true that if research achievement is deemed important in selection for a post, the possession of an intercalated degree is a useful marker.

Our findings support much of what has previously been said about the propensity of Oxbridge graduates and qualifiers with optional intercalated degrees to choose medicine and pathology, and to take up academic posts. In our cohorts they obtained more postgraduate qualifications than other graduates, were more likely to concentrate in the teaching hospital centres where they graduated, and were less likely to enter general practice. They also rated more highly than other qualifiers the importance and usefulness of research and their competence in dealing with it (see Chapter 15). In our questionnaire we did not specifically ask for people's opinions about intercalated degrees; bearing in mind that our enquiry was more general, we found very few respondents who spontaneously, to quote Smith (1986), 'speak very positively of the experience' or who, as in Wakeford *et al.*'s (1985) study, reported that undergraduate research had a positive influence on them.

Positive proof of the value of intercalated degrees is hard to obtain, even on research grounds; and the possibility that some intercalated degrees might actually have a more general educational value, although this is even less measurable than research, is surely not such a dread prospect as the National Audit Office seemed to think. Wakeford *et al.* (1985) noted that 'the most frequently reported positive influence on the decision to follow a research career was intrinsic motivation'. Common sense, if nothing else, suggests that a well-directed year, spent at a receptive stage, is likely to further the development of research interests and insights, or kill them altogether. All the evidence, including that from our surveys, indicates that those who are offered intercalated degree courses and elect to take them up do tend to appear on their subsequent track record as a worthwhile group of people within the more academic realms of medicine.

5 Career progress

Postgraduate examinations

We looked at the postgraduate qualifications obtained by doctors who qualified in 1974 and in 1977, since by the time we concluded our surveys these doctors were sufficiently advanced in their careers to have most of their experience of these examinations behind them (Parkhouse and Ellin 1989).

Table 5.1 shows the numbers and percentages of respondents obtaining UK qualifications. Table 5.2 gives the same information for other qualifications: 81.8 per cent of 1974 respondents and 90.1 per cent of 1977 respondents were known to hold one or more postgraduate qualifications, 78.8 per cent and 75.7 per cent respectively of all known qualifiers in these two years.

For UK qualifications the 1974 and 1977 qualifiers were similar. Almost a quarter of all respondents held the DRCOG; almost 20 per cent had the MRCP and a similar proportion had the MRCGP. An FRCS was held by about 10 per cent of respondents and the DCH by rather fewer. The next most commonly held examinations were the FFARCS and the MRC Psych. The numbers of university higher degrees were somewhat lower among 1977 qualifiers than those of 1974, and the same was true of overseas qualifications and enabling examinations such as the ECFMG, LMCC, FLEX and VQE.

SEX DIFFERENCES

Table 5.3 shows that most of the principal UK qualifications were held by higher percentages of men than women, the outstanding examples being the FRCS and, to a lesser extent, university higher degrees. The qualifications held by considerably higher percentages of women than men were the MRC Psych, DRCOG, and the Family Planning Certificate.

Table 5.1 UK qualifications (percentages of respondents to one or more questionnaires)[a]

	1974 qualifiers		*1977 qualifiers*	
Qualification	*no.*	*%*	*no.*	*%*
MRCP 1	554	24.4	660	22.1
MRCP 2	440	19.4	551	18.4
FRCS 1	263	11.6	336	11.2
FRCS 2	234	10.3	303	10.1
MRCOG 1	75	3.3	81	2.7
MRCOG 2	51	2.2	58	1.9
FFARCS 1	152	6.7	213	7.1
FFARCS 2	121	5.3	164	5.5
FRCR 1	63	2.8	91	3.0
FRCR 2	57	2.5	75	2.5
MRC Path 1	50	2.2	80	2.7
MRC Path 2	65	2.9	68	2.3
MRC Psych 1	99	4.4	132	4.4
MRC Psych 2	94	4.1	113	3.8
MRCGP	411	18.1	588	19.7
MFCM	12	0.5	6	0.2
DRCOG	516	22.7	703	23.5
DCH	204	9.0	226	7.6
DA	50	2.2	59	2.0
DO	12	0.5	20	0.7
DLO	1	–	3	0.1
DMRD/T	30	1.3	36	1.2
DTM&H	14	0.6	19	0.6
DPM	6	0.3	1	–
DIH	7	0.3	4	0.1
Dip Av Med	14	0.6	7	0.2
FP Cert	96	4.2	84	2.8
MD	126	5.5	59	2.0
MSc/MPhil	43	1.9	39	1.3
Phd/DPhil	22	1.0	9	0.3
MS/MChir	17	0.7	13	0.4
MCh Orth	5	0.2	2	0.1
Other qualifications (UK)	80	3.5	99	3.3

Note: a Numbers show doctors holding one or more of each qualification
Source: Parkhouse and Ellin 1989

Table 5.2 Other qualifications (percentages of respondents to one or more questionnaires)

Qualification	*1974 qualifiers* *no.*	*%*	*1977 qualifiers* *no.*	*%*
ECFMG	38	1.7	25	0.8
LMCC	39	1.7	24	0.8
FLEX	26	1.1	15	0.5
VQE	15	0.7	6	0.2
FRACP	14	0.6	3	–
FRACS	2	–	2	–
FRCPC	21	0.9	11	0.4
FRCSC	7	0.3	2	–
US Boards Internal Medicine	10	0.4	6	0.2
Other US boards	22	1.0	12	0.4
CCFPC	6	0.3	4	–
MRNZCGP	7	0.3	1	–
Other foreign qualifications	64	2.8	50	1.7
FDS RCS	9	0.4	9	0.3
Other non-medical	6	0.3	3	–

Source: Parkhouse and Ellin 1989

MEDICAL SCHOOL DIFFERENCES

Table 5.4 gives a grouping of medical schools and shows numbers of main hospital specialty qualifications obtained by 1974 and 1977 qualifiers combined. Oxford and Cambridge, Wales, and Belfast are shown separately, although the numbers in these groups are often small. It is clear that the MRCP and FRCS were obtained by higher percentages of qualifiers from the London medical schools than from Scotland or the English provincial schools. Scotland, Wales, and Belfast tended to produce more qualifiers who obtained the MRCOG, and Scotland and Oxford showed relatively high percentages with the MRC Path; Scotland, the English provincial schools and Belfast showed higher percentages of holders of the MRC Psych than London, Oxford or Wales.

Table 5.3 Main qualifications by sex (percentages of respondents to one or more questionnaires)

	1974 qualifiers		*1977 qualifiers*	
Qualification	*Men*	*Women*	*Men*	*Women*
MRCP	20.5	16.2	20.5	14.1
FRCS	13.4	1.8	14.0	2.2
MRCOG	2.2	2.3	1.9	2.0
FFARCS	6.0	3.6	5.8	4.9
FRCR	2.3	2.9	2.7	2.1
MRC Path	3.0	2.5	2.1	2.5
MRC Psych	3.7	5.2	2.9	5.5
MFCM	0.5	0.7	0.1	0.3
MRCGP	18.2	17.8	19.8	19.5
DRCOG	21.6	25.7	21.3	28.0
DCH	7.6	12.7	6.4	10.0
FP Cert	2.8	8.0	1.8	4.8
MD	7.1	1.3	2.6	0.7
PhD/DPhil	1.1	0.5	0.4	0.0
MS/MChir	0.8	0.7	0.6	0.1

Source: Parkhouse and Ellin 1989

Between individual medical schools, the ranges were considerable: for the MRCP, from 6.4 per cent of respondents (Dundee, 1977) to 37.7 per cent (the Middlesex Hospital, 1977); for the FRCS, from 1.8/1.9 per cent of respondents (Oxford/Leeds, 1977) to 19.2 per cent (Charing Cross Hospital, 1977). The range for the FFARCS was from 1.1 per cent of respondents (Royal Free Hospital, 1974) to 13.9 per cent (King's College Hospital, 1974). For the MRCOG, FRCR, MRC Path and MRC Psych, several medical schools had no holders, while others had from 6.6 per cent (MRCOG, St George's Hospital, 1974) to 9.4 per cent (MRC Psych, Dundee 1974). For both 1974 and 1977 qualifiers, the medical schools which came within the top three for percentages of respondents holding various examinations were: MRCP, Oxford; FRCS, Charing Cross Hospital; MRCOG, St George's Hospital; FFARCS, St Mary's Hospital; FRCR, Guy's Hospital; MRC Path, St George's Hospital; MRC Psych, Birmingham. In the bottom three medical schools for both 1974 and 1977 were: MRCP, Sheffield/Dundee; FRCS, Aberdeen; MRCOG, Charing Cross Hospital; FRCR, Charing Cross Hospital.

Table 5.4 Main qualifications in hospital specialties – medical school differences (1974 and 1977 qualifiers combined: percentages of respondents to one or more questionnaires)

Medical school group	*MRCP*	*FRCS*	*MRCOG*	*FFARCS*	*FRCR*	*MRC Path*	*MRC Psych*	*No. of respondents*
Scotland	14.3	9.7	2.6	5.2	2.0	3.4	4.7	1,084
English provincial[a]	14.1	8.5	1.6	5.8	2.0	1.7	4.7	1,696
Oxford/Cambridge[b]	30.2	7.5	1.9	4.7	2.8	3.8	0.9[c]	106
London	25.1	12.3	1.9	5.6	2.7	2.8	3.1	2,036
Wales	14.5	7.7	3.4	2.9	5.8	1.9	1.9	207
Belfast[d]	18.3	9.2	4.6	5.3	5.3	1.5	6.1	131

Notes: a 1977 data included Nottingham and Southampton
b Four Cambridge (clinical) qualifiers only (1977)
c One person
d 1977 data only
Source: Parkhouse and Ellin 1989

Table 5.5 Time of passing main specialty examinations (numbers of qualifiers: 1974 and 1977 combined)

Exam	*Years since qualifying*													*Total with known dates*	*Exam. dates not given*	*Total*
	1	*2*	*3*	*4*	*5*	*6*	*7*	*8*	*9*	*10*	*11*	*12*	*13*			
MRCP	1	164	354	180	95	35	14	9	3	3	1	1	–	860	131	991
FRCS	–	–	4	161	178	73	22	16	6	1	2	1	–	464	73	537
MRCOG	–	–	–	1	27	26	16	10	8	–	–	–	–	88	21	109
FFARCS	–	–	1	59	89	45	23	12	4	1	3	–	–	237	48	285
FRCR	–	–	–	–	7	23	21	19	14	8	2	4	–	98	34	132
MRC Path	–	–	1	–	–	22	28	20	17	3	3	2	–	96	37	133
MRC Psych	–	–	–	41	53	27	14	13	7	1	2	–	1	159	48	207
All above exams	1	164	360	442	449	251	138	99	59	17	13	8	1	2,002	392	2,394

Source: Parkhouse and Ellin 1989

Table 5.6 MRCP: numbers of respondents working in various specialties (1974 qualifiers in 1987 and 1977 qualifiers in 1986)[a]

Respondents	*Medicine*	*Neurology*	*Rheumatology*	*Dermatology*	*Genito-urinary medicine*	*Geriatrics*	*Paediatrics*	*Other medical specialties*	*Haematology*	*Other pathology*	*Radiology/radiotherapy*
SHO/Registrar	8	1	1	2	0	1	8	1	1	0	4
SR/Consultant/Principal	129	11	12	24	4	33	46	5	37	13	12
Academic	62	9	6	4	2	3	33	5	7	1	9
Other/unknown	15	3	2	5	0	1	10	2	1	0	2
Abroad	26	1	2	2	0	2	6	2	0	2	1
Total	240	25	23	37	6	40	103	15	46	16	28
% of *men* with MRCP	31.7	3.6	2.4	3.4	0.9	4.4	9.6	1.6	4.9	1.9	2.8
% of *women* with MRCP	11.8	0.5	3.2	6.4	0.0	4.5	17.3	1.8	5.9	1.4	4.1
Nos holding other PG qualifications	97	13	7	6	1	9	54	7	34	11	22
% of no. in specialty	40	52	30	16		23	52	47	74	69	79
Nos holding intercalated degrees	55	5	5	10	3	8	22	5	16	6	7
% of no. in specialty	23	20	22	27	50	20	21	33	35	38	25

Table 5.6 continued

	Other hospital specialties	*General practice*	*Community medicine*	*Other/ unknown*	*Unemployed*	*Total*	*(% of 4,387 respondents)*	*Men*	*(% of 3,010 respondents)*	*Women*	*(% of 1,377 respondents)*
SHO/Registrar	17	0	0	0	0	44		31		13	
SR/Consultant/Principal	54	117	2	3	0	502		396		106	
Academic	15	2	3	2	0	163		129		34	
Other/unknown	7	23	15	18	13	117		68		49	
Abroad	6	7	2	8	2	69		51		18	
Total	99	149	22	31	15	895	(20.4)	675	(22.4)	220	(16.0)
% of *men* with MRCP	11.4	16.3	1.6	3.0	0.4	100					
% of *women* with MRCP	10.0	17.8	5.0	5.0	5.5	100					
Nos holding other PG qualifications	90	99	16	18	9	493		374		119	
% of no. in specialty	91	66	73	58	60	55.1		55.4		54.1	
Nos holding intercalated degrees	30	26	5	10	5	218		174		44	
% of no. in specialty	30	17	23	32	33	24.4		25.8		20.0	

Note: a Percentages based on very small numbers are not shown
Source: Parkhouse and Ellin 1989

TIME OF PASSING EXAMINATIONS

Table 5.5 shows the year in which each of the principal examinations in the hospital specialties was passed minus the calendar year of qualification. This is an indication of the time taken to pass the examinations, but it is imprecise since the month of qualification varied widely, as did the month in which examinations were passed. Nevertheless, the table shows that the peak period for obtaining the MRCP was three years after qualifying, for the FRCS, MRCOG, FFARCS and MRC Psych five years after qualifying, and later for other examinations. The table gives numbers for 1974 and 1977 qualifiers combined; at the time of our latest surveys the 1977 group had been qualified for nine years, so the numbers in the table for ten to thirteen years, which are included for interest, relate to 1974 qualifiers only.

WHAT DO EXAMINATION HOLDERS DO?

Tables 5.6 to 5.12 deal successively with the individual major examinations in the hospital specialties, showing what the holders of these qualifications who replied to us in 1986 or 1987 were doing at or about April of those years respectively. Qualifiers of 1974 and 1977, men and women, are shown together in order to maximize the numbers in each cell of the tables, which thus represent the varying progress of doctors nine and thirteen years after qualifying and after passing examinations at different times from leaving medical school (Table 5.5).

MRCP

The first column of Table 5.6, headed 'Medicine', includes general medicine, chest medicine, cardiology, gastroenterology, endocrinology, nephrology, clinical pharmacology and infectious diseases.

The great majority of doctors with the MRCP had progressed beyond the SHO/registrar stage, the exception being those in hospital work outside the medical specialties. Altogether, 60 per cent of the MRCP holders were working in medicine or a medical specialty, including paediatrics and haematology; 27 per cent were working in 'medicine', 17 per cent were in general practice, 16 per cent in various other hospital specialties, and almost 10 per cent in paediatrics. Of the women with the MRCP, over 17 per cent were working in paediatrics, almost 18 per cent in general practice, and only less than 12 per cent in 'medicine'. Considerable numbers of MRCP holders also possessed other postgraduate qualifications especially, as would be expected, those working in other hospital specialties, general practice, and community medicine. Almost 25 per cent of respondents with the MRCP had optional intercalated degrees from their undergraduate years.

Of the 129 respondents who were senior registrars or consultants in 'medicine', 111 were working in general medicine, six in chest medicine, 3 in cardiology, 3 in gastroenterology, 2 in endocrinology, 2 in nephrology, 1 in clinical pharmacology, and 1 in infectious diseases.

FRCS

Table 5.7 shows that 21 per cent of FRCS holders were in the SHO/registrar grades, compared to 5 per cent of MRCP holders (Table 5.6). Twelve of the nineteen respondents in plastic surgery (63 per cent) were still in these grades and proportions were also high among those in paediatric surgery and other (non-surgical) hospital specialties where in both cases the total numbers were small.

Of respondents with the FRCS 84 per cent were working in general surgery or a surgical specialty. Of the men, 35 per cent were working in general surgery and/or urology, and 19 per cent in orthopaedics. Among the relatively few women with the FRCS, 22 per cent were working in ophthalmology and 19 per cent in general surgery/urology. Only twenty-one holders of the FRCS (4.4 per cent) were in general practice, and only ten (2.1 per cent) in obstetrics and gynaecology. Postgraduate qualifications other than an FRCS were the most commonly held by those working in obstetrics and gynaecology, radiology and radiotherapy, general practice, or in general surgery. About 13 per cent of respondents with the FRCS had taken an optional undergraduate intercalated degree. Of the sixty-seven senior registrars or consultants in surgery/urology, fifty were working in general surgery, sixteen in urology and one in specialized surgery of the colon.

Table 5.7 FRCS: numbers of respondents working in various specialties (1974 qualifiers in 1987 and 1977 qualifiers in 1986)[a]

Respondents	*Surgery/ urology*	*Accident & emergency*	*ENT*	*Neuro-surgery*	*Ophthal-mology*	*Ortho-paedics*	*Paediatric surgery*	*Plastic surgery*	*Cardiac surgery*	*Medical specialties*	*Obstetrics & gynaecology*	*Radiology/ radiotherapy*
SHO/registrar	30	3	3	4	3	22	4	12	3	2	3	5
SR/consultant/principal	67	15	26	8	32	46	2	2	10	0	5	6
Academic	29	0	1	0	0	10	0	1	0	1	2	0
Other/unknown	17	2	2	0	3	4	0	2	0	0	0	0
Abroad	16	1	2	1	3	5	0	2	4	0	0	0
Total	159	21	34	13	41	87	6	19	17	3	10	11
% of *men* with FRCS	34.8	4.3	7.0	3.0	7.7	18.9	0.9	3.9	3.9	0.5	2.3	2.5
% of *women* with FRCS	18.8		9.4	0	21.9	12.5	6.3	6.3	0		0	0
Nos holding other PG qualifications	59	2	7	2	22	17	2	4	6	1	10	10
% of no. in specialty	37	10	21	15	34	20	33	21	35		100	91
Nos holding intercalated degrees	21	4	2	2	4	13	1	2	2	0	2	1
% of no. in specialty	13	19	6	15	10	15	17	11	12	0	20	9

Table 5.7 continued

Respondents	*Other hospital specialties*	*General practice*	*Community medicine*	*Other/ unknown*	*Non-medical*	*Dental*	*Unemployed*	*Total*	*(% of 4,387 respondents)*	*Men*	*(% of 3,010 respondents)*	*Women*	*(% of 1,377 respondents)*
SHO/registrar	5	0	1	1	0	0	0	101		93		8	
SR/consultant/principal	0	11	0	0	0	4	0	234		221		13	
Academic	0	0	0	2	0	1	0	47		41		6	
Other/unknown	0	7	1	6	0	0	4	48		45		3	
Abroad	0	3	0	3	1	1	0	42		40		2	
Total	5	21	2	12	1	6	4	472	(10.7)	440	(14.6)	32	(2.3)
% of *men* with FRCS	0.9	4.8	0.2	2.3	0.2	1.4	0.7	100					
% of *women* with FRCS		0		6.3	0	0		100					
Nos holding other PG qualifications	2	11	0	3	0	6	1	165		155		10	
% of no. in specialty	40	52	0	25	0	100	25	35.0		35.2		31.3	
Nos holding intercalated degrees	0	4	1	1	1	0	0	61		60		1	
% of no. in specialty	0	19		8		0	0	12.9		13.6		3.1	

Note: a Percentages based on very small numbers are not shown
Source: Parkhouse and Ellin 1989

Table 5.8 MRCOG: numbers of respondents working in various specialties (1974 qualifiers in 1987 and 1977 qualifiers in 1986)[a]

Respondents	*Obstetrics & gynaecology*	*Other hospital specialties*	*General practice*	*Community medicine*
SHO/registrar	8	0	0	0
SR/consultant/principal	38	1	7	0
Academic	14	0	0	0
Other/unknown	9	2	2	3
Abroad	8	0	1	1
Total	77	3	10	4
% of *men* with MRCOG	83.8		7.4	2.9
% of *women* with MRCOG	60.6		15.2	6.1
Nos holding other PG qualifications	46	1	5	3
% of no. in specialty	60		50	75
Nos holding intercalated degrees	7	0	0	0
% of no. in specialty	9.1			

Note: a Percentages based on very small numbers are not shown
Source: Parkhouse and Ellin 1989

MRCOG

Table 5.8 shows that 84 per cent of men with the MRCOG were working in obstetrics and gynaecology but only 61 per cent of women, proportionately more of whom were in general practice, community medicine, or were unemployed. Of those working in the specialty 60 per cent had other higher qualifications, most commonly the DRCOG; a relatively small number of MRCOG holders had optional intercalated degrees.

Other/ unknown	*Non-medical*	*Unemployed*	*Total (% of 4,387 respondents)*	*Men (% of 3,010 respondents)*	*Women (% of 1,377 respondents)*
0	0	0	8	5	3
0	0	0	46	34	12
0	0	0	14	9	5
0	0	5	21	11	10
1	1	0	12	9	3
1	1	5	101 (2.3)	68 (2.3)	33 (2.4)
		2.9	100		
		9.1	100		
1	1	2	59	44	15
			58.4	64.7	45.5
0	0	1	8	6	2
			7.9	8.8	6.1

FFARCS

Over 80 per cent of women with the FFARCS, and over 90 per cent of men were working in anaesthetics (Table 5.9).

MRC Psych

Almost all of the men with the MRC Psych, and 86 per cent of the women, were working in some branch of the specialty (Table 5.10).

Table 5.9 FFARCS: numbers of respondents working in various specialties (1974 qualifiers in 1987 and 1977 qualifiers in 1986)[a]

Respondents	*Anaesthetics*	*Other hospital specialties*	*General practice*	*Other/ unknown*	*Non-medical*
SHO/registrar	12	0	0	0	0
SR/consultant/principal	172	1	8	0	0
Academic	17	1	0	1	0
Other/unknown	11	2	2	3	1
Abroad	21	0	0	0	0
Total	233	4	10	4	1
% of *men* with FFARCS	92.3	1.0	4.1	1.5	
% of *women* with FFARCS	81.8	3.0	3.0	1.5	
Nos holding other PG qualifications	64	3	2	0	1
% of no. in specialty	27	75	20		
Nos holding inter-calated degrees	27	1	0	0	0
% of no. in specialty	11.6				

Note: a Percentages based on very small numbers are not shown
Source: Parkhouse and Ellin 1989

Of the 121 senior registrars or consultants in psychiatry, 73 were working in general/adult psychiatry, 27 in child and adolescent psychiatry, 6 in psychogeriatrics, 7 in psychotherapy, 5 in forensic psychiatry, 2 in mental handicap and 1 in neuropsychiatry.

FRCR

Table 5.11 shows that proportionately more women than men with the FRCR were working in radiotherapy; almost 80 per cent of the FRCR holders working in radiology and radiotherapy held additional postgraduate qualifications, and a relatively high proportion had optional intercalated degrees. There were no FRCR holders working in general practice.

Unemployed	*Total (% of 4,387 respondents)*		*Men (% of 3,010 respondents)*		*Women (% of 1,377 respondents)*	
0	12		9		3	
0	181		140		41	
0	19		16		3	
7	26		12		14	
1	22		17		5	
8	260	(5.9)	194	(6.4)	66	(4.8)
0.5	100					
10.6	100					
3	73		57		16	
38	28.1		29.4		24.2	
0	28		21		7	
	10.8		10.8		10.6	

MRC Path

Table 5.12 shows that only two respondents with the MRC Path, working in haematology, were in the SHO/registrar grades. Of women respondents with the MRC Path, 35 per cent were working in microbiology, the next most popular specialties among women MRC Path holders being histopathology and haematology. There were no women working in chemical pathology. The most popular specialties among men with the MRC Path were histopathology and haematology. Additional postgraduate qualifications, and optional intercalated undergraduate degrees, were most commonly held by those working in haematology, chemical pathology and microbiology. All the respondents with the MRC Path were working in some branch of pathology.

Table 5.10 MRC Psych: numbers of respondents working in various specialties (1974 qualifiers in 1987 and 1977 qualifiers in 1986)[a]

Respondents	*Psychiatry*	*General practice*	*Community medicine*	*Other/ unknown*	*Unemployed*	*Total (% of 4,387 respondents)*		*Men (% of 3,010 respondents)*		*Women (% of 1,377 respondents)*	
SHO/registrar	10	0	0	0	0	10		3		7	
SR/consultant/ principal	121	1	0	1	0	123		73		50	
Academic	19	0	0	0	0	19		15		4	
Other/unknown	13	1	1	1	6	22		9		13	
Abroad	15	0	0	0	1	16		11		5	
Total	178	2	1	2	7	190	(4.3)	111	(3.7)	79	(5.7)
% of *men* with MRC Psych	99.1	0	0.9	0	0	100					
% of *women* with MRC Psych	86.1	2.5	0	2.5	8.9	100					
Nos holding other PG qualifications	77	2	0	2	3	84		. 51		33	
% of no. in specialty	43				43	44.2		45.9		41.8	
Nos holding inter-calated degrees	27	2	1	1	0	31		17		14	
% of no. in specialty	15					16.3		15.3		17.7	

Note: a Percentages based on very small numbers are not shown
Source: Parkhouse and Ellin 1989

Table 5.11 FRCR: numbers of respondents working in various specialties (1974 qualifiers in 1987 and 1977 qualifiers in 1986)[a]

Respondents	*Radiology*	*Radiotherapy*	*Other hospital specialties*	*Unemployed*	*Total (% of 4,387 respondents)*	*Men (% of 3,100 respondents)*	*Women (% of 1,377 respondents)*
SHO/registrar	1	2	0	0	3	3	0
SR/consultant	85	13	1	0	99	70	29
Academic	6	4	0	0	10	7	3
Other/unknown	2	1	0	2	5	3	2
Abroad	3	2	0	0	5	2	3
Total	97	22	1	2	122 (2.8)	85 (2.8)	37 (2.7)
% of *men* with FRCR	82.4	15.3	1.2	1.2	100		
% of *women* with FRCR	73.0	24.3		2.7	100		
Nos holding other PG qualifications	78	17	1	2	98	71	27
% of no. in specialty	80	77			80.3	83.6	73.0
Nos holding inter-calated degrees	16	4	0	0	20	13	7
% of no. in specialty	16	18	0	0	16.4	15.3	18.9

Note: a Percentages based on very small numbers are not shown
Source: Parkhouse and Ellin 1989

Table 5.12 MRC Path: numbers of respondents working in various specialties (1974 qualifiers in 1987 and 1977 qualifiers in 1986)[a]

Respondents	*Pathology*	*Histo-pathology*	*Micro-biology*	*Chemical pathology*	*Haematology*
SHO/registrar	0	0	0	0	2
SR/consultant	3	29	18	6	29
Academic	2	12	2	1	4
Other/unknown	5	1	3	0	1
Abroad	0	1	0	0	0
Total	10	43	23	7	36
% of *men* with MRC Path	8.0	37.5	11.4	8.0	29.6
% of *women* with MRC Path	8.1	27.0	35.1	0	27.0
Nos holding other qualifications	1	15	16	4	33
% of no. in specialty	10	35	70	57	92
Nos holding inter-calated degrees	1	9	6	3	12
% of no. in specialty	10	21	26	43	33

Note: a Percentages based on very small numbers are not shown
Source: Parkhouse and Ellin 1989

DISCUSSION

The *plurality* of postgraduate examinations does not diminish, for sure, as training supposedly improves. Allowing for a miscellaneous group of 'other' qualifications, at least forty separate UK examinations had been passed by our respondents. The number of examinations passed averages out at 2.0 each for all known qualifiers of 1974 and 1.9 each for all those of 1977. Why so many of these examinations are taken, and what use is made of them, can partly be seen from this analysis, but altogether the state of affairs remains hard to understand fully (Parkhouse 1988).

Forensic pathology	Immunology	Blood transfusion	Total (% of 4,387 respondents)	Men (% of 3,010 respondents)	Women (% of 1,377 respondents)
0	0	0	2	0	2
1	2	2	90	65	25
0	0	0	21	16	5
1	0	0	11	6	5
0	0	0	1	1	0
2	2	2	125 (2.8)	88 (2.9)	37
1.1	2.3	2.3	100		
2.7	0	0	100		
2	2	1	74	52	22
			59.2	59.1	59.5
0	0	0	31	29	2
0	0	0	24.8	33.0	5.4

The *specificity* of the examinations varies considerably. Of our respondents who had the MRCP, 60 per cent of those who replied to our surveys in 1986 and 1987 were working in medicine or a medical specialty at those times; 84 per cent of those with the FRCS were working in general surgery or a surgical specialty. For the other major examinations in the hospital specialties, the percentages of working in the specialty concerned were extremely high. An exception to this general statement is that only 61 per cent of women with the MRCOG were working in obstetrics and gynaecology, a fact which may well illustrate the difficulties encountered by women in this specialty, although domestic commitments probably accounted for much of what may be a temporary loss.

The *variability* in the numbers of graduates taking examinations is shown by some striking medical school differences. These suggest a range of traditions and styles in the selection and counselling of students in regard to their attitudes and approach to their future careers. One question is whether these variations make a difference to career prospects; a more important question is whether there are any good reasons why they should.

The *perceived necessity* of certain examinations has varied over the years. Many senior psychiatrists hold the MRCP (or FRCP) but among 151 of our 1974 and 1977 qualifiers who were known to have become senior registrars and/or consultants in psychiatry, only 8 held the MRCP. Similarly only 8 of 101 of our respondents with the MRCOG also had the FRCS. Haematology is currently betwixt the MRCP and the MRC Path.

The perceived value or necessity of diploma examinations is difficult to assess. For example, the numbers of our 1977 respondents obtaining these diplomas ranged from 703 with the DRCOG to 3 with the DLO and 1 with the DPM. Many such diploma examinations are taken by potential entrants into general practice as is, of course, the MRCGP.

The *sufficiency* of individual examinations in the currently chaotic hospital scramble for a place in the sun, or at least in the security of the NHS, is obviously questionable when 40 per cent of our respondents who were working in general medicine had at least one postgraduate qualification in addition to the MRCP, and 37 per cent of those working in general surgery or urology had at least one qualification additional to their fellowships in surgery. The existence of similar examinations in the same specialty, particularly surgery, continues to provoke strong views and prejudices, and some confusion in non-medical and foreign circles. Included in Tables 5.1 and 5.2 are twenty-one 1974 qualifiers who had more than one FRCS and three who had both British and Irish FFARCS. Among 1977 qualifiers were fifty-eight with more than one FRCS, four with more than one primary FRCS, three with both British and Irish FFARCS and two with both MRCPs, and two with two FRCPCs. The superimposition of specialized fellowships in specific branches of surgery is a further topic of vigorous debate (Delamothe 1988).

The *international utility* of UK qualifications does not show strongly from these data. On emigration, language difficulties may be less in some specialties than others — the 'microbes don't speak Dutch' view of the 1970s; in some specialties work abroad may be lucrative. But only one of our respondents with the MRC Path was working abroad, only 4 per cent of those with the FRCR and 8 per cent of those with the FFARCS, compared with 8 per cent of those with the MRCP and the MRC Psych, 9 per cent of those with the FRCS and 12 per cent of those with the MRCOG. Some of the older-established examinations may be more valued abroad, unless now overshadowed by nationalism, and since this chapter is concerned with examinations it does not relate how many doctors were successfully practising abroad in these various specialties without the recognized UK examination.

The *career significance* of different examinations varies greatly between specialties.

In anaesthetics, data from the College of Anaesthetists show that the number of candidates from UK medical schools who passed the final FFARCS in the academic year 1981/82 was 158 — a fairly average year for the time. Those doctors would have qualified at various times prior to 1981, as shown by Table 5.5. Our figures suggest that about 5.4 per cent of the qualifiers in 1974 and in 1977 obtained the FFARCS. Assuming this to be the same for other cohorts, and relating the percentages passing to the times after graduation and the sizes of the graduating classes, the number of doctors who would have been expected from our data to pass the FFARCS in 1981/82 works out at about 160. These doctors, who passed the FFARCS in 1981/82, would be seeking consultant appointments some years later. The numbers of paid consultant anaesthetists appointed in the NHS in England and Wales were 101 in 1983/84, 88 in 1984/85, and 112 in 1985/86. To this average of 100 an allowance must be made for appointments in Scotland, where the number of consultants is about 14 per cent of that in England and Wales, and to some academic posts, making perhaps an approximate total of 120-5 vacancies a year at consultant level in Great Britain. Of our respondents, about 18 per cent of those with the FFARCS were working in anaesthetics abroad or were not working in anaesthetics. The remaining 82 per cent, from the above calculations, would represent about 125-30 doctors. This suggests a reasonable fit between the numbers of doctors passing the FFARCS in the early 1980s and the numbers of consultant vacancies three or four years later, but with two provisos: the numbers of consultant appointments in recent years have allowed a high rate of expansion in the specialty and this must clearly continue if a bottleneck is to be avoided; and the assumption has to be made that a certain number of doctors with the FFARCS work abroad, or do not work in anaesthetics from choice rather than because consultant posts are not available.

Similar calculations for psychiatry, based on the percentages of our respondents obtaining the MRC Psych at various times after qualifying, would suggest that in the early 1980s the number of passes would be about 120 a year. The Royal College of Psychiatrists data show that the actual number of passes among graduates of UK medical schools in the academic year 1981/82 was 159 — again, a fairly average year. It may be that the numbers of 1974 and 1977 qualifiers passing the examination were lower than average, or that there are late passes not captured by our data. The numbers of paid consultants appointed in England and Wales in all the psychiatric specialties for the years 1983/84 to 1985/86 average 114 a year. Making an allowance again for appointments held in Scotland and to academic posts, the approximate number of vacancies would be 140, which once more corresponds fairly well with the number of examination passes when some allowance is made for holders of the examinations who practise abroad or do not work in the specialty. The same proviso, particularly that regarding consultant expansion, must again be made.

A significant difference between anaesthetics and psychiatry is that in recent years the numbers of UK candidates passing the final MRC Psych have shown a much greater increase than have the numbers passing the final FFARCS. A prospective analysis of the relationship to career opportunities, for more recent qualifiers than those of 1974 and 1977, might therefore show less similarity between the two specialties.

For the FRCS, data from the Royal Colleges show that the total number of passes in the final examinations in London, Edinburgh and Glasgow in the early 1980s was about 360 a year. From our data it is possible to estimate the number of doctors who pass more than one of these examinations, although not necessarily in the same year; allowing about 15 per cent for this double-counting, the number of individuals obtaining one or more fellowships in surgery would be a little over 300 a year. This fits reasonably well with our figures. The numbers of paid consultants appointed in the NHS in England and Wales in all the surgical specialties averaged 131 between 1983/84 and 1985/86. Even a generous allowance for appointments in Scotland and to academic posts would leave the number of vacancies, perhaps 160-70 a year, far below the number of British graduates passing an FRCS. The figures in this survey show that 84 per cent of our respondents with the FRCS were working in the surgical specialties but of these respondents eighty-four (18 per cent) were still in the SHO/registrar grades, forty-one (9 per cent) were in academic posts, many of which were of the research-registrar type, thirty (6 per cent) were in 'other' types of surgical post and thirty-four (7 per cent) were working in surgery abroad. Thus about 77 per cent of those with the FRCS were, at the time of our latest surveys, working in surgery in the UK and if the number of career vacancies is, at best, about 60 per cent of the number of doctors obtaining an FRCS examination each year, the implication is clear — and well known. One important factor is that over recent years general surgery has been a non-expanding specialty; another is the relatively limited range of career options available to holders of the FRCS, compared to those with the MRCP.

These differences in career significance can be seen by relating career choices and examination passes in a specialty, as percentages of qualifying doctors, to NHS career openings in the specialty as percentages of all career openings. Available Department of Health tables and publications (DHSS 1987a) show numbers of consultants appointed and numbers of new admissions to general practice; openings in community medicine and community health can be roughly assessed from numbers and whole-time equivalents of doctors in post. For 1974 qualifiers, career choices for anaesthetics and psychiatry were 4.2 and 3.5 per cent of all choices at the pre-registration stage, and 6.2 and 4.7 per cent of choices six years later (Table 3.13). The FFARCS and MRC Psych were known to be held by 5.3 and 4.1 per cent of respondents respectively, in each case thus falling between the levels of interest at one and seven years after qualifying, although our MRC Psych figures appear to be low compared to Royal College data. NHS career openings in anaesthetics and psychiatry in 1985/86 can be estimated from England and Wales data as approximately 5.1 and 5.9 per cent of all NHS career openings. This suggests a closer relationship for anaesthetics than for psychiatry, unless in percentage terms the number of career outlets in psychiatry is greater outside than within the NHS. In general surgery and the surgical specialties, career choices declined from 15.6 per cent after leaving medical school to 11.1 per cent six years later, while 10.3 per cent of respondents were known to hold an FRCS. However, career openings in all branches of surgery since 1985/86 appeared to represent only 6.4 per cent of all career prospects in the NHS in England and Wales.

6 Career progress

Internal migration – who goes where?

MOVEMENT DURING TRAINING

We studied this among 1974 qualifiers (Parkhouse and Ellin 1990a). Included in the questionnaire sent to them in 1985 was a section asking how many times people had moved 'in the course of training', over various distances and including moves abroad. We specified that moves for short locums and moves of less than fifteen miles should not be included, thus eliminating most movements between hospitals within a city. A total of 1,830 questionnaires were returned (78.7 per cent, not allowing for those deceased or untraceable). In seventy-nine cases the questions on movement were not answered; the results, shown as percentages of respondents to the 1985 questionnaire, thus potentially underestimate the amount of movement, although it is likely that in many cases no entry signified no movement.

Table 6.1 shows the aggregate numbers of moves made by men and women respondents. Since the options given were to circle 0, 1, 2, 3 or '4 or more' moves, the numbers greater than 4 represent minima. Without allowing for this the 'average' number of moves was a little over three; the most common pattern among men was three moves and among women, one.

Table 6.2 shows range of movement. Women moved less commonly and less frequently than men. Of all respondents, 48 per cent were known to have made at least one move of 15-20 miles; rather fewer had made longer moves and 28 per cent were known to have been abroad at least once. Among those making only one move the commonest picture was a move of 15-50 miles (5 per cent of men and 8 per cent of women respondents) or one trip abroad (3 per cent of men and 4 per cent of women respondents). There was a very large variety of combinations of moves, the commonest being two or three moves of 15-50 miles, or one move of 15-50 miles plus a move of 50-100 or 100-200 miles.

Table 6.1 Total number of moves, including abroad (1974 respondents in 1985)

No. of moves	*No. of respondents*	*%*	*Men (%)*	*Women (%)*
0	194	10.6	8.6	15.7
1	303	16.6	14.6	21.6
2	283	15.5	15.2	16.3
3	311	17.0	17.7	15.3
4+	238	13.0	13.9	10.8
5+	178	9.7	9.9	9.2
6+	109	6.0	7.0	3.1
7+	71	3.9	4.9	1.2
8+	33	1.8	2.3	0.6
9+	17	0.9	1.0	0.8
10+	7	0.4	0.5	–
11+	6	0.3	0.4	0.2
12+	1	0.1	0.1	–
?	79	4.3	3.9	5.3

Table 6.3 shows frequency of moves in relation to the latest career choice (1985) of respondents. In surgery (including surgical specialties), obstetrics and gynaecology, and paediatrics, over 50 per cent of respondents were known to have moved four or more times, and over 40 per cent had done so in anaesthetics and medicine (including the medical specialties). In general practice, radiotherapy and non-medical career choices fewer than 30 per cent of respondents were known to have moved four or more times. In all specialties except psychiatry and community medicine, where no difference was seen, fewer women than men had moved four or more times. Some differences in this respect were large; in paediatrics only 34 per cent of men, compared to 65 per cent of women had moved fewer than four times; in obstetrics and gynaecology these figures were 38 and 65 per cent, and in surgery 39 and 78 per cent but many of the relatively small number of women concerned had chosen surgical specialties rather than general surgery or orthopaedics. In the small, miscellaneous category of 'other medical' career choices movement was frequent and considerably greater among men than women.

Table 6.2 Number of moves over distances indicated (1974 qualifiers in 1985: percentages)

		No. of moves				
Distance		*0*	*1*	*2*	*3*	*4+*
15-50 miles	Men	46	22	13	8	6
	Women	51	24	11	6	3
	Total	48	23	13	7	5
50-100 miles	Men	61	18	11	4	3
	Women	69	15	7	3	1
	Total	63	17	10	3	3
100-200 miles	Men	63	15	11	5	2
	Women	66	17	9	2	1
	Total	63	16	10	4	2
200+ miles	Men	69	13	6	4	3
	Women	69	17	7	1	2
	Total	69	14	6	3	3
Abroad	Men	67	19	6	2	2
	Women	74	15	4	1	–
	Total	69	18	6	2	2

Table 6.4 gives a grouping of medical schools and shows a tendency for movement to be more frequent among London qualifiers than those of Scotland, Wales and the provinces. Oxford is shown separately; although there were only thirty-six respondents (80 per cent) the frequency of movement is notable.

Individual medical schools showed wider variation. Among qualifiers from Glasgow, Liverpool, Leeds and Manchester over 70 per cent reported fewer than four moves, whereas 50 per cent or fewer did so from the Middlesex, St Bartholomew's and St George's. For all medical schools except the Royal Free and University College Hospital there were fewer women than men who reported four or more moves. Some of the sex differences in frequency of movement within London medical schools appeared large in percentage terms but the numbers of women respondents were small. Also, differences in the amount of movement among qualifiers from individual medical schools were partially explained by differences in the sex ratio of qualifiers and the proportions of career choices for surgery and general practice.

Table 6.3 Number of moves by latest career choice (1974 qualifiers in 1985)

No. of moves	*Medicine*	*Paediatrics*	*Surgery*	*Obstetrics & gynaecology*	*GP ± other*	*Psychiatry*	*Community medicine*	*Pathology*	*Anaes-thetics*	*Radiology*	*Radio-therapy*	*Other medical*	*Non-medical*
0-3	56.1	43.1	42.2	46.3	66.1	66.5	55.5	65.2	54.2	67.3	68.2	38.5	73.3
4+	40.5	53.4	54.6	53.7	29.1	32.4	38.2	31.9	44.8	30.6	27.3	61.5	13.3
?	3.3	3.5	3.2	0.0	4.8	1.1	6.3	2.9	1.0	2.0	4.5	0.0	13.3

Table 6.4 Number of moves by medical school group (1974 qualifiers in 1985)

Medical school group	*0–3 moves*			*4 or more moves*		
	men	*women*	*total*	*men*	*women*	*total*
Scotland	58.8	65.2	60.8	36.8	30.4	34.8
English provincial	63.4	74.2	67.0	32.9	22.0	29.3
Oxford	32.3	40.0[a]	33.3	64.5	60.0[a]	63.9
London	51.6	66.8	55.2	44.5	25.7	40.1
Wales	56.3	65.0	58.8	39.6	30.0	36.8

Note: a Five respondents only

LOCATIONS OF SENIOR REGISTRAR AND CONSULTANT POSTS

Among the doctors qualifying in 1974 and 1977, up to and including their latest replies to us in 1987 and 1986 respectively, there were 1,188 respondents who were known to have been NHS senior registrars, and 603 who were known to have been NHS consultants. Tables 6.5 and 6.6 show the locations of the first substantive appointments in these grades.

From Table 6.5, 86 per cent of the Queen's University, Belfast, qualifiers who had been senior registrars had held these posts in Northern Ireland; 48 per cent of Scottish qualifiers had held their senior registrar posts in Scotland and 43 of University of Wales College of Medicine qualifiers in Wales. Of 516 London medical school qualifiers known to have been senior registrars, 273 (53 per cent) had held their senior registrar posts in one of the four Thames regions. Only fifteen of these posts were described as being outside Greater London, but others would certainly include rotations.

The only individual British medical schools from which over 50 per cent of qualifiers had held senior registrar posts in their own region were Glasgow, Nottingham and Manchester. Only two of fifty-seven senior registrars from Bristol were in the South Western Region; two of twenty-six from Oxford were in the Oxford region and one of thirteen from Southampton was in Wessex.

Of the 1974 and 1977 respondents appointed to senior registrar posts in Scotland 79 per cent were from Scottish medical schools, 75 per cent of those appointed in the Thames regions were from London medical schools and 42 per cent of those appointed in Wales were from the University of Wales College of Medicine. The balance or imbalance between numbers of qualifiers becoming senior registrars from a medical school and numbers of senior registrar appointments in the region of the medical school is complex. For example of fifty-eight respondents appointed to senior registrar posts in the Northern region, only fourteen were Newcastle qualifiers and of forty-six appointed in the South Western region, only two were Bristol qualifiers. However, fifty-seven Bristol qualifiers among our respondents obtained senior registrar posts in various regions while the South Western region itself appointed only forty-six of all our respondents as senior registrars, whereas although thirty-one of our Newcastle qualifiers became senior registrars the Northern region appointed fifty-eight of our respondents as senior registrars.

Table 6.6 shows consultant posts. Of Queen's University, Belfast, qualifiers with consultant posts, 95 per cent held these posts in Northern Ireland; 51 per cent of Scottish qualifiers worked in Scotland and 50 per cent of University of Wales College of Medicine qualifiers worked in Wales. Of the 234 London medical school qualifiers known to have become consultants, 86 (37 per cent) held these posts in one of the Thames regions, 59 of the 86 posts being in Greater London.

As with the distribution of senior registrar appointments there were wide variations between medical schools and regions. Only one of eighteen Dundee qualifiers becoming consultants was in Tayside, only one of twenty-two Bristol qualifiers was in the South Western region and none of ten Oxford qualifiers was in the Oxford region; but 45-50 per cent of the qualifiers from Newcastle, Manchester and Glasgow who had become consultants held their consultant posts in the region of their medical school.

Altogether, the extent to which qualifiers from each medical school are spread across the regions can be studied from Table 6.6, as can the sources from which regions drew their British-qualified consultants. A crude numerical balance sheet, derived from Table 6.6, is shown in Table 6.7. This is of interest concerning the 'internal market' debate about distribution of medical school places and, through the Joint Planning Advisory Committee, of senior registrar posts. It is also of some interest concerning the self-sufficiency principle of medical school intake in relation to NHS needs, but only so far as the hospital

Table 6.5 Respondents known to have held senior registrar appointments (1974 and 1977 qualifiers)[a]

	Location of first substantive senior registrar post										
Medical school	*Northern*	*Yorkshire*	*Trent*	*East Anglia*	*Wessex*	*Oxford*	*South Western*	*West Midlands*	*Mersey*	*North Western*	*Thames regions*
Birmingham	2	1	6	2	2	2	2	16	0	5	0
Bristol	1	3	6	3	1	3	2	7	5	7	0
Leeds	2	10	2	1	1	3	3	4	4	2	0
Liverpool	1	3	4	0	1	1	1	6	20	5	0
Manchester	3	1	2	1	2	1	2	0	2	27	3
Newcastle	14	4	2	2	0	0	0	2	1	1	0
Oxford	2	3	1	3	0	2	4	1	1	0	0
Sheffield	2	2	12	0	1	1	4	0	1	5	0
Nottingham	1	0	5	1	0	1	0	0	0	0	0
Southampton	1	0	3	1	1	1	2	0	0	1	1
London medical schools	12	13	36	24	33	22	19	23	13	17	15
Aberdeen	6	3	2	0	2	0	1	1	0	3	1
Dundee	2	1	3	0	1	3	2	1	1	1	0
Edinburgh	4	2	5	3	0	0	1	2	1	3	0
Glasgow	4	1	3	0	3	0	2	0	2	6	0
Wales	0	2	4	0	0	0	1	2	0	3	0
Belfast	1	1	1	0	0	0	0	0	0	1	0
Total	58	50	97	41	48	40	46	65	51	87	20

Table 6.5 continued

Medical school	Location of first substantive senior registrar post Greater London	North Scotland	Grampian	Tayside	Lothian	West Scotland	Wales	Northern Ireland	Not known	Total
Birmingham	7	0	0	0	2	2	2	0	2	53
Bristol	13	0	0	0	0	2	1	1	2	57
Leeds	7	0	0	0	0	0	1	0	1	41
Liverpool	6	0	0	0	0	1	3	0	1	53
Manchester	7	0	0	0	0	1	1	0	0	53
Newcastle	3	0	0	0	1	0	1	0	0	31
Oxford	6	0	1	0	1	1	0	0	0	26
Sheffield	4	0	0	0	0	1	0	0	0	33
Nottingham	1	0	0	0	0	0	0	0	0	9
Southampton	2	0	0	0	0	0	0	0	0	13
London medical schools	258	0	2	0	5	6	8	0	10	516
Aberdeen	2	0	4	3	1	6	3	1	0	39
Dundee	2	0	0	7	5	0	1	0	4	34
Edinburgh	11	0	1	4	15	6	2	1	1	62
Glasgow	6	0	2	1	4	46	2	1	1	84
Wales	10	0	0	0	0	1	18	0	1	42
Belfast	0	0	0	0	1	0	0	36	1	42
Total	345	0	10	15	35	73	43	40	24	1,188

Note: a Figures are numbers of doctors
Source: Parkhouse and Ellin 1990a

Table 6.6 Respondents known to have held consultant appointments (1974 and 1977 qualifiers)[a]

	Location of first substantive consultant post										
Medical school	*Northern*	*Yorkshire*	*Trent*	*East Anglia*	*Wessex*	*Oxford*	*South Western*	*West Midlands*	*Mersey*	*North Western*	*Thames regions*
Birmingham	1	2	1	1	0	2	0	13	1	3	2
Bristol	0	3	4	0	0	1	1	6	0	0	2
Leeds	1	5	3	1	0	0	0	3	1	0	0
Liverpool	6	2	1	0	0	0	0	2	7	2	2
Manchester	2	1	1	2	3	0	0	3	1	13	1
Newcastle	11	4	3	0	0	1	0	3	0	1	1
Oxford	2	2	3	1	0	0	1	0	1	0	0
Sheffield	2	1	4	0	0	0	1	2	0	3	1
Nottingham	0	0	0	1	0	0	0	0	0	0	0
Southampton	1	0	1	0	2	0	0	0	0	1	0
London medical schools	10	9	21	10	16	11	17	26	4	12	27
Aberdeen	3	1	1	1	1	1	1	0	1	0	2
Dundee	1	0	5	0	2	0	0	1	2	1	0
Edinburgh	2	2	2	1	0	1	0	4	1	4	2
Glasgow	2	3	1	0	4	0	1	3	0	3	1
Wales	0	2	2	0	0	1	0	2	1	1	1
Belfast	0	0	0	0	0	0	0	0	0	0	0
Total	44	37	53	18	28	18	22	68	20	44	42

Table 6.6 continued

	Location of first substantive consultant post									
Medical school	*Greater London*	*North Scotland*	*NE Grampain*	*Tayside*	*Lothian*	*West Scotland*	*Wales*	*Northern Ireland*	*Not known*	*Total*
Birmingham	1	1	0	1	1	0	1	0	0	31
Bristol	2	0	0	0	0	1	0	1	1	22
Leeds	0	0	0	0	1	0	0	0	0	15
Liverpool	2	0	1	0	0	0	1	0	0	26
Manchester	2	0	0	0	0	0	0	0	0	29
Newcastle	0	0	0	0	0	0	0	0	0	24
Oxford	0	0	0	0	0	0	0	0	0	10
Sheffield	2	0	0	0	1	0	0	0	0	17
Nottingham	0	0	0	0	0	0	0	0	0	1
Southampton	0	0	0	0	0	0	0	0	0	5
London medical schools	59	1	0	0	2	3	4	0	2	234
Aberdeen	1	1	4	1	2	5	1	0	0	27
Dundee	1	0	1	1	1	1	1	0	0	18
Edinburgh	2	0	3	3	9	6	2	1	0	45
Glasgow	1	0	3	4	1	27	0	0	0	54
Wales	3	0	0	0	0	0	13	0	0	26
Belfast	1	0	0	0	0	0	0	18	0	19
Total	77	3	12	10	18	43	23	20	3	603

Note: a Figures are numbers of doctors
Source: Parkhouse and Ellin 1990a

Table 6.7 Distribution of consultant appointments (1974 and 1977 qualifiers)[a]

Medical school/region	*Qualifiers from the medical school becoming consultants (in all NHS regions)*	*Consultants appointed in the region (from total of column 1)*	*'Excess regional demand' for consultants*
Birmingham/West Midlands	31	68	+37
Bristol/South Western	22	22	0
Leeds/Yorkshire	15	37	+22
Liverpool/Mersey	26	20	-6
Manchester/North Western	29	44	+15
Newcastle/Northern	24	44	+20
Sheffield and Nottingham[b]/Trent	18	53	+35
Southampton[b]/Wessex	5	28	+23
Oxford/Oxford	10	18	+8
London/Thames	234	119	-115
Aberdeen/Grampian and North Scotland	27	15	-12
Dundee/Tayside	18	10	-8
Edinburgh/Lothian	45	18	-27
Glasgow/West Scotland	54	43	-11
Cardiff/Wales	26	23	-3
Belfast[b]/Northern Ireland	19	20	+1

Notes: a Figures are numbers of doctors
b 1977 qualifiers only
Eighteen consultants appointed were in East Anglia
Location of three consultant appointments is unknown
Source: Parkhouse and Ellin 1990a

sector is concerned. The table does not, of course, show numbers of overseas qualified doctors appointed to consultant posts, nor does it show how many British qualified doctors become consultants abroad. For regions, it relates to fairly recent consultant appointments; for medical schools it tends to show what the situation was, and what changes might have been good, at the time when these doctors qualified in 1974 and 1977. Some of the changes have come about; Nottingham and Southampton did not have medical schools in 1974 and Cambridge and Leicester have begun producing doctors since 1977. The general picture is of concentration of medical education in London and Scotland.

Table 6.8 Appointments in relation to region of medical school

Year of qualifying		*Senior registrars in region of medical school*		*Consultants in region of medical school*		*Consultants in region of senior registrarship*		*Senior registrar and consultant in region of medical school*	
1974	Men	195/464	42%	103/339	30%	132/287	46%	65/287	23%
	Women	42/110	38%	24/70	34%	39/63	62%	20/63	32%
1977	Men	195/438	45%	59/143	41%	74/130	57%	40/130	31%
	Women	76/151	50%	28/48	58%	34/42	81%	23/42	55%
1974 and 1977 combined	Men	390/902	43%	162/482	34%	206/417	49%	105/417	25%
	Women	118/261	45%	52/118	44%	73/105	70%	43/105	41%

Source: Parkhouse and Ellin 1990a

Table 6.8 shows that about 44 per cent of the 1974 and 1977 qualifiers who were known to have become senior registrars and 36 per cent of those known to have become consultants held their posts in the region of their medical school. Both senior registrar and consultant appointments were in the medical school region in 28 per cent of cases. For 1977 qualifiers, both men and women, senior registrar and consultant posts were more commonly held in the region of the medical school than for 1974 qualifiers. In both cohorts, women were more likely than men to become consultants in the region of their medical school and considerably more likely to hold senior registrar and consultant appointments in that region. This is consistent with the finding that 70 per cent of women respondents held consultant posts in the same region as their senior registrar appointments. Possible explanations abound; women are often less able to move freely from region to region than men, and the fact that they do tend to move less is seen throughout this chapter. A directly or indirectly related factor is that women doctors are more highly concentrated in the specialties which show less movement during training. The high proportion of women becoming consultants in the region where they have been senior registrars may also indicate a high level of competence and achievement at the senior registrar level. The 1977 qualifiers who had become consultants by the time of their latest reply to us in 1986 would certainly include the majority of high-fliers, who might be more likely to achieve senior registrar and consultant posts in the region of their medical school. Our studies of some individual specialties (Chapters 12 and 13), based on the same cohorts of respondents, indicate that in anaesthetics the women who became senior registrars and consultants, although fewer than men, made slightly more rapid progress, but the reverse was true in psychiatry.

RELATIONSHIP TO FAMILY HOME

We found that 38 per cent of 1974 respondents and 44 per cent of 1977 respondents had family homes in the region of their clinical medical school. Of those who had become consultants, 16 per cent and 28 per cent respectively had both a family home and a consultant post in the region of their clinical medical school. The higher percentages among 1977 qualifiers are largely due to the inclusion of Northern Ireland, where 98 per cent of respondents from Queen's University, Belfast, had family homes and 89 per cent of those with consultant posts had both their family home and their consultant post in that region.

For both cohorts combined, 53 per cent of University of Wales College of Medicine respondents had family homes in Wales, 52 per cent of those from Scottish medical schools had family homes in Scotland and 43 per cent from London medical schools had family homes in Greater London or one of the Thames regions. Percentages of respondents with family homes in the region of individual medical schools varied widely: 93 per cent from Glasgow University, 59 per cent from Aberdeen and 55 per cent from Newcastle, to 13 per cent from Bristol, 12 per cent from Oxford, 5 per cent from Leeds and 3 per cent from Dundee. Glasgow University medical school also showed a high percentage (43 per cent) of respondents with both family home and consultant post in the West of Scotland.

The tendency to move to and settle in a family region was less notable than the tendency to remain in, or return to the region of the medical school. Among respondents with family homes outside the region of their clinical medical school, only 13 per cent held senior registrar posts in the region of their family home; 17 per cent of those with consultant posts of known location held these posts in the region of their family home, but 26 per cent held their consultant posts in the region of their clinical medical school. However, only 12 per cent of consultant posts held by Scottish qualifiers with family homes outside their medical school region were in Scotland, compared to 28 per cent of consultant posts held in London and the Thames regions by London medical school qualifiers with family homes outside these regions.

COMMENT

Assuming that postgraduate education aims to train appropriate numbers of specialists effectively, with safety to the patient, and to a high standard, it can scarcely fail to be unsatisfactory to expect most of these doctors to struggle for the jobs they need piecemeal. It has been clear for years (Parkhouse and Darton 1979) that many young doctors would welcome better organized postgraduate training programmes, and this is especially true when repeated movement brings no benefit or when there are compelling reasons to stay in one place. As one respondent wrote from Canada:

> The main early attraction was a structured residency training programme in my chosen specialty. Once accepted in the

> programme I did not have to move . . . the programme director is responsible for ensuring appropriate variety of experience and training.

But it must also be stressed that freedom of movement has its advantages during training. The possibility of building up experience by applying for jobs of different types as they become available, and of progressing at a pace to suit one's aptitude and inclinations, gives flexibility to a system which otherwise could easily become too formal and unforgiving. For those who have to move for domestic or other reasons this flexibility should make it possible to continue training with little detriment, and the same should apply to those who wish to spend time working in the Third World or developing other interests at a creative time of life. In practice, it often happens that the criteria for promotion and the attitudes of appointment committees fail even to approximate to this ideal.

Freedom of movement is important. Trainees should always have the chance to apply to centres and regions of their choice although, as with vocational training for general practice, market forces will inevitably produce some local bias. The aim of better planning is emphatically not to restrict the graduates of each medical school to the self-contained postgraduate training opportunities in their own region. But it is important for each medical centre, and each region, to have appropriate numbers of staff in each grade, including senior and experienced trainees; and it is important for each region to be able to develop its full potential for providing good training at various levels, rather than allowing senior registrar posts to remain concentrated in some regions to the detriments of others (Parkhouse *et al.* 1987).

The problem of reconciling good planning with individual freedom, and good training with good patient care, is not easily solved. The emphasis in the NHS has been too much on lack of planning, and on patient care which is too heavily dependent on junior staff. This is illustrated by our data on movement during training. A shift towards more thoughtful planning of each trainee's programme, with tolerance towards domestic and other claims upon time and ability, is long overdue.

7 Career progress

International movement

Some of the changes in medical emigration since the early analysis of the Willink Committee in 1957, which concentrated mainly on the colonial medical service and missionary work, have been referred to in Chapter 1. Easy movement around the world has progressively declined since the 1960s for various reasons. The situation in 1978 was reviewed by Glaser in a report for the United Nations Organization (Glaser 1978) in which he considered 'the range of personal motives, economic incentives and social influences that govern the decisions of the individual to emigrate — to be used as a basis for policy making'. Doctors do still go abroad, and we made a detailed study of this among the 1974 qualifiers, to whom we sent a specifically worded questionnaire for the purpose in 1987 (Parkhouse and Parkhouse 1990). We have less detailed information about 1977, 1980 and 1983 qualifiers.

THE 1974 QUALIFIERS

Of 2,272 respondents, 1,660 (73.1 per cent) were men and 612 (26.9 per cent) were women; 601 of the men (36.2 per cent) and 176 of the women (28.8 per cent) were known to have been abroad at some time, giving a combined total of 777 (34.2 per cent). By medical school groups, the numbers who had been abroad are shown in Table 7.1

The percentages of respondents abroad in each year from 1975 are shown in Table 7.2, for three medical school groups and the combined total. Table 7.3 shows the numbers of respondents known to be abroad, by year, from individual medical schools.

The total number deduced to be abroad at the time of their last reply (i.e. those who had not returned to work in the UK) was 278 (12.2 per cent). Of those still abroad, ninety-nine were consultants or the equivalent, forty-eight were engaged in academic work, and twenty-nine were in training posts including

Table 7.1 Respondents known to have been abroad by 1987, by medical school group (1974 qualifiers)

Medical school group	*No. in cohort*	*Been abroad*	*%*
English provincial and Wales	815	251	30.8
Scotland	481	178	37.0
London	976	348	35.7

retraining — for example, a doctor who had changed direction to become a Fellow in Medical Administration. Eighty were working in general practice, including doctors in New Zealand, Australia and Canada, where family practice is often combined with specialist work in the local hospital. Twenty-two were doing other kinds of work: four were in the pharmaceutical industry, three were ship's doctors, three were directing health care programmes and four were doing general missionary work in the Third World; one was editor of a medical journal, two were in company medicine, one was in the Canadian Navy, one was travelling, and three were unemployed.

Of the fifty-eight women currently abroad, forty-eight were married or divorced, and forty-three of these mentioned their husband's work as the reason for going abroad. The single women, as in this country, had advanced more easily in their careers: one was an associate professor, four were full-time consultants, one was a principal in general practice, and one — a doctor who had spent much of her time travelling — was in a training grade. One was director of a Third World health programme, one a director in the pharmaceutical industry, and one a ship's doctor. Among the married and divorced women, all of whom had children, seven were in academic work and seven were consultants, three of whom were working part-time. Eighteen were in general practice, including five part-time, eleven were in training grades, one was in the pharmaceutical industry, one was the editor of a medical journal, one was working in the Third World, and two were unemployed. Some of these women felt that being abroad because of a husband's work was an additional obstacle to their own careers, but one who was working part-time as an anaesthetist in Canada, where her husband was researching into immunology, was glad that she

Table 7.2 Percentage of respondents abroad in each year, by medical school group (1974 qualifiers)

Medical school group	*No. in cohort*	*Percentages* 1975	*1976*	*1977*	*1978*	*1979*	*1980*	*1981*	*1982*	*1983*	*1984*	*1985*	*1986*	*1987*
English provincial and Wales	815	2.3	6.8	9.6	11.8	13.5	13.1	13.7	14.4	13.4	13.9	13.0	12.8	11.5
Scotland	481	6.7	10.4	13.9	15.2	16.2	17.5	17.5	15.4	16.6	15.6	15.6	15.8	14.8
London	976	4.3	9.5	11.0	13.2	14.6	15.7	13.3	13.9	13.4	12.1	12.3	11.3	10.8
Total	2,272	4.1	8.7	11.1	13.1	14.5	15.1	14.4	14.4	14.1	13.5	13.3	12.8	11.9

Table 7.3 Number of respondents abroad in each year, by individual medical school (1974 qualifiers)

Medical school	*No. in school*	*1975*	*1976*	*1977*	*1978*	*1979*	*1980*	*1981*	*1982*	*1983*	*1984*	*1985*	*1986*	*1987*
Birmingham	116	4	10	14	18	20	17	22	24	18	18	17	17	13
Bristol	88	2	5	9	12	15	13	11	10	12	14	13	12	10
Leeds	74	1	5	9	11	12	9	8	6	8	10	8	7	7
Liverpool	110	1	4	5	8	12	12	10	10	11	10	12	15	14
Manchester	143	5	10	11	15	13	16	16	15	16	18	17	14	13
Newcastle	77	1	3	4	3	7	8	9	12	9	8	7	7	6
Oxford	45	1	6	9	10	11	9	9	13	11	10	7	7	7
Sheffield	75	4	9	11	13	14	13	15	16	13	14	14	13	14
Wales	87	0	3	6	6	6	10	12	11	11	11	11	12	10
Provinces/Wales total	815	19	55	78	96	110	107	112	117	109	113	106	104	94
Aberdeen	93	11	13	14	13	16	20	19	13	14	12	12	14	14
Dundee	64	3	5	9	12	14	15	14	12	10	12	12	14	11
Edinburgh	142	8	14	19	23	22	24	22	22	26	22	24	21	19
Glasgow	182	10	18	25	25	26	25	29	27	30	29	27	27	27
Scotland total	481	32	50	67	73	78	84	84	74	80	75	75	76	71

Table 7.3 continued

Medical school	*No. in school*	*1975*	*1976*	*1977*	*1978*	*1979*	*1980*	*1981*	*1982*	*1983*	*1984*	*1985*	*1986*	*1987*
Charing Cross	38	2	7	6	5	6	5	7	6	5	3	5	4	4
Guy's	113	7	7	11	16	19	20	15	13	14	12	9	9	9
King's College	79	3	5	10	14	15	13	14	16	15	11	14	14	12
The London	111	1	7	9	12	16	21	16	15	18	19	19	15	15
Middlesex	81	4	6	5	8	9	14	9	8	8	6	4	4	3
Royal Free	87	5	8	8	9	13	10	5	7	8	7	10	9	8
St Bart's	80	7	12	15	13	18	14	16	18	16	17	13	13	14
St George's	61	1	3	3	5	7	9	6	6	3	3	5	5	3
St Mary's	81	3	8	12	12	9	9	9	10	10	10	8	7	8
St Thomas'	78	2	12	11	16	14	15	13	14	14	14	15	12	12
UCH	103	6	11	11	11	8	13	12	15	13	10	11	11	10
Westminster	64	1	7	6	8	8	10	8	8	7	6	7	7	7
London total	976	42	93	107	129	142	153	130	136	131	118	120	110	105

Table 7.4 Respondents abroad and their intentions, by medical school group (1974 qualifiers)

Medical school group	*No. of respondents*	*% ever having been abroad*			*% intending to stay abroad permanently*	*% intending 'definitely not' to practise in UK*	*% living abroad at last reply*
		men	*women*	*total*			
Scotland	481	41.4	26.9	37.0	14.3	9.1	16.4
English provincial and Wales	815	31.4	29.4	30.8	10.6	4.7	10.6
London	976	37.5	29.3	35.7	9.9	6.8	11.6
Total	2,272	36.2	28.8	34.2	11.1	6.5	12.2

Note: *Differences* between Scottish medical schools and other medical schools combined are statistically significant (chi-square) for:

- Intention to remain abroad permanently $p<0.05$
- Intention definitely not to practise in UK $p<0.05$
- Number of doctors abroad at last reply $p<0.01$

had 'a job that will travel, and job-share allows for family commitment'. Eight women were abroad because of being married to foreign nationals: 'came for holiday and got married', wrote one in Australia, and another was a paediatrician in Nigeria, where her husband had been born. Four were born abroad: one was a lecturer in medicine in Hong Kong, one born in Malaysia was researching into molecular biology in Singapore, one born in Taiwan was an assistant professor in the USA, and the fourth was a Fellow in haematology also in the USA.

Patterns of movement

We looked at the total duration of time spent abroad by each doctor; whether the move was time-limited or permanent; whether the final intention of staying abroad was 'definite', 'possible', or 'undecided'; the number of moves to one country only or between countries; the reasons for going, and the countries moved to.

Table 7.4 shows that among Scottish qualifiers there were significantly higher percentages than from other medical school groups of respondents indicating that they regarded themselves as being abroad permanently rather than on a time-limited basis, of respondents declaring their intention of 'definitely not' practising ultimately in the UK, and of respondents living abroad at the time of their latest reply. In general, the percentages of men having been abroad were higher than those of women. This difference was small among qualifiers from English provincial medical schools and the University of Wales College of Medicine, larger among London qualifiers and largest among Scottish qualifiers where, although the percentage of women respondents having been abroad was actually the lowest for any of the three medical school groups, the total percentage of men and women having been abroad was the highest. Only from the Royal Free Hospital medical school was the actual number of women who had been abroad higher than the number of men who had done so.

Table 7.5 shows that when the total lengths of time spent abroad are added up for each respondent, over 40 per cent of those having been abroad had spent more than three years out of the UK. Some of those still abroad at their latest reply had been abroad for ten years or more. The commonest length of time to have spent abroad was one to two years (24.7 per cent of those having been abroad). From Scottish medical schools, compared with English and Welsh medical schools, significantly fewer

Table 7.5 Total amounts of time spent abroad (1974 qualifiers)

Medical school group	*Percentage of all respondents who had been abroad* less than 1 year	up to 3 years	over 3 years	*Total number having been abroad*
Scotland	12.3	49.4	50.6	178
English provincial and Wales	23.9	59.4	40.6	251
London	23.3	61.2	38.8	348
Total	21.0	57.9	42.1	777

Note: *Differences* between Scottish medical schools and other medical schools combined are statistically significant (chi-square) for:
- Numbers abroad for less than one year $p<0.01$
- Numbers abroad for more than three years $p<0.05$

respondents had been abroad for less than one year, and significantly more had spent over three years abroad.

Among individual medical schools, over 50 per cent of respondents from Oxford had been abroad, over 45 per cent from the Middlesex Hospital, and over 40 per cent from Bristol, Birmingham, Charing Cross, King's College Hospital and St Thomas'. Fewer than 20 per cent of respondents had been abroad from the University of Wales College of Medicine and St George's Hospital, fewer than 25 per cent from Liverpool and Newcastle, and fewer than 30 per cent from Leeds, Manchester, Sheffield, the Royal Free Hospital and University College Hospital. The highest proportions actually abroad at the time of their latest reply were from the medical schools of Glasgow (19.8 per cent, St Bartholomew's Hospital (17.5 per cent), Sheffield (17.3 per cent) and Dundee (17.2 per cent). The lowest proportions were from St George's Hospital (4.9 per cent), Newcastle (7.8 per cent), Bristol (8.0 per cent), and Guy's Hospital (8.0 per cent).

Of all respondents who had been abroad, 76.8 per cent had visited one country only, although this might include living and/or working in more than one location within the same coun-

Table 7.6 Countries to which respondents had been, from all medical schools combined (1974 qualifiers)

Countries	*No. of respondents*	*% of 777 respondents having been abroad*
Australia	157	20.2
Canada	148	19.0
USA	131	16.9
EC	106	13.6
Far East	83	10.7
New Zealand	74	9.5
Africa (excluding RSA)	69	8.9
Middle East	47	6.0
Europe (non-EC)	35	4.5
West Indies, etc.	34	4.4
South Africa	31	4.0
India	25	3.2
Near East	24	3.1
South America, etc.	20	2.6
Ship's doctor	16	2.1
Arctic/Antarctic	5	0.6
Unspecified	9	1.2

try; 17.6 per cent had visited two countries, 4.1 per cent had been to three and 1.4 per cent to four or more countries.

Table 7.6 shows that Australia was the most frequently visited country, followed by Canada, the USA and EC countries. Only 6 of 178 respondents (3.4 per cent) from Scottish medical schools who had been abroad had gone to Far Eastern countries, compared with 42 of 348 London qualifiers (12.1 per cent) and 35 of 251 qualifiers (13.9 per cent) from English provincial medical schools and the University of Wales College of Medicine.

Reasons for going abroad

Table 7.7 shows the frequency with which respondents ticked one or more of various reasons listed in the questionnaire for going abroad. Taking all medical schools together, the commonest reasons were adventure, travel, or vacation — ticked by 30.8 per cent of those who had been abroad, but sometimes combined

Table 7.7 Reasons given for going abroad by respondents, from all medical schools combined (1974 qualifiers)

Reasons given	*No. of respondents*	*% of 777 respondents having been abroad*
Adventure/travel/vacation	239	30.8
Better life-style/living conditions	187	24.1
Better career prospects/work-style	172	22.1
Visiting fellowship/rotation/ secondment	160	20.6
Better financial prospects	145	18.7
View to permanent emigration	139	17.9
Dissatisfaction with NHS	110	14.2
Missionary work/Third World medicine	85	10.9
Spouse's career	79	10.2
Dissatisfaction with life in UK	76	9.8
Dissatisfaction with career prospects at home	75	9.7
Better research prospects	73	9.4
Armed Forces	69	8.9
VSO	3	0.4

with other reasons. It was outstandingly the commonest reason given by qualifiers from London medical schools (35.3 per cent); but among Scottish qualifiers (21.3 per cent) it was actually the third commonest reason, visiting fellowships or secondments and better career prospects being given higher priority.

Only 8 of 178 Scottish qualifiers (4.5 per cent) who had been abroad gave missionary work or Third World medicine as a reason, compared with 29 of 251 qualifiers (11.6 per cent) from English provincial medical schools and the University of Wales College of Medicine, and 48 of 348 London qualifiers (13.8 per cent). In addition, Voluntary Service Overseas (VSO) was specifically indicated by only three respondents, all from London medical schools.

Thirty-six qualifiers from English provincial medical schools and the University of Wales College of Medicine (14.3 per cent), and twenty from Scottish medical schools (11.2 per cent) gave as a reason for going abroad a spouse's career or marriage to a foreign national, compared with only twenty-three London qualifiers (6.6 per cent).

Comment — where, when and why

Periods spent abroad may be short- or long-term, voluntary or unwilling, and the reasons for going and returning may be positive or negative. Each doctor has a unique combination of reasons and we can identify only some of the more common factors in motivation.

Where

Most emigrants went to Australia, New Zealand, Canada and the USA. In Europe, both within and beyond the EC, numbers were small: for example members of the Armed Forces in West Germany, doctors working for WHO in Geneva or in the American Hospital in Paris, or a Norwegian returning home.

In the Near East, which we defined as countries bordering on the Mediterranean, there were, for example, doctors working in Beersheba in Israel and in the Armed Forces in Cyprus. In the Middle East, doctors were mainly working short-term in Saudi Arabia. In the Far East, including New Guinea and the Solomon Islands, we found doctors in Hong Kong (in the University and in the Armed Forces), and doing missionary work in Papua and Borneo. With India we included Sri Lanka, the Seychelles and Mauritius, and also Nepal, Bangladesh and Pakistan. We divided Africa into the Republic of South Africa, where doctors went for career advancement, and the rest of the continent, which included the homelands and where the work was mainly missionary. South and Central America and the South Atlantic included work in the Falklands, St Helena and Ascension Islands; in the Arctic and Antarctic doctors took part in expeditions. From the West Indies and Bermuda a consultant, after eight years' stay, wrote 'I came for six months on my way to see the world but Bermuda is very difficult to leave'.

When

When does 'permanent' become 'forever'? One emigrant classed herself as permanent but was 'keeping an eye open for return for family reasons'. Missionary work may be on a three-year rolling contract so it is permanent with a question mark; post-independence commitment (e.g. tropical medicine research in the Gambia) depends on politics. Temporary visits may be for VSO; secondments during career progress, e.g. on a senior registrar rotation; by personal arrangement, e.g. locums in Australia, or expeditions; or moving with a spouse, e.g. in the Armed Forces. This may lead to staying on, or returning as a permanent emigrant to the country visited:

> I will put a time limit on getting a job in UK or returning to South Africa.

> I will go if prospects for medicine don't improve in UK.

> Dissatisfaction with NHS would make me go.

Temporary visits often include planned travel time: one doctor worked in Iran so as to be able to travel to Afghanistan, India and the Far East; another worked for two years in Africa, having spent a year travelling there. There are short visits to centres of excellence to lecture and to learn, including one to Hong Kong to learn acupuncture; temporary work in the Forces included one doctor loaned by the British to the Sultan of Brunei's Armed Forces.

Why

Some reasons are above and beyond voluntary control:

> A knowledge that God in Christ has done everything for me and that I owe it to Him to do what He wants — hence when He said 'Pakistan', I came.

The often unwilling emigration of women doctors married to husbands in the Armed Forces is interesting, and has echoes of Empire days except that now the women want to find work and the children don't have to be sent home for education:

> My career has been severely curtailed by marrying into the Armed Forces and electing to accompany my husband on all his tours. While I am always able to find employment of some form within medicine, I frequently take jobs I do not particularly want; I am not able to build up any seniority of significance. I would strongly advise any woman in medical school today to think long and hard about her prospective life partner's job commitments and likely demands on her own time and stability within a community.

> MRC Psych not fully accepted — I need two years' neurology full-time on call. My advice is to find out exactly what the prospects of finding work abroad are, and being aware of what the various specialties accept and recognize. (Respondent working as a registrar equivalent in a long-stay psychiatric hospital in West Germany)

> I have chosen to follow my husband in the Armed Forces, so am unable to follow a career plan despite personal motivation; part-time training is very limited and domestic responsibilities important, so I don't allow myself choice but take what's going.

> Having been moved round the world with my husband in the Armed Forces my career is in shambles: experience not accepted for a vocational training certificate.

> It is difficult for a wife to find medical work within the army medical service. Pay is not on par with male colleagues and with two children I have now returned to UK working as a civilian for army while husband is on tour.

> The emigration issue has over-taken me and we are moving permanently to the USA. This is entirely to further my husband's career, and I go with him reluctantly. I don't know if I shall ever work again. (Not in Armed Forces)

A common *negative reason for emigration* is dissatisfaction with conditions at home:

> I have no objection to any aspect of England except the weather — I enjoy an outdoor life.

So do a lot of us who live in Britain. One doctor started as an anatomy demonstrator in 1975, and after his training in surgery was either unemployed or worked as a locum until he left in exasperation for Hong Kong in 1986, where he is now a lecturer/consultant. A physician who returned from Johns Hopkins, Baltimore, 'for ideological reasons and commitment to NHS', will go back:

> The NHS has changed since the late 1970s to provide a very second-rate service to the nation (both to the patients and medical profession). It is unlikely that the NHS will ever now be able to compete with its European let alone American

> equivalents, given the apathy of the Nation and its doctors, and the British complacency for second best.

A consultant paediatrician in Sydney took the post when offered because there were none in the UK:

> Morale and service expectations of senior registrars, with minimal thoughts for 'training', were major reasons for going.

A family practitioner in British Columbia, who is also a member of staff at the local hospital, regretted

> the ennui in government and medical circles to elevate the UK above Third World status for preventable diseases such as rubella.

Similarly in the field of research into public health:

> I consider AIDS to be the most important health problem this decade and want to work in an area of research related to it.

At an earlier stage the lack of planned career opportunities in the UK is deplored, especially in oversubscribed specialties:

> I became set on the surgical rails from which it was difficult to change. I was good at surgery but not prepared to devote endless hours making statistics work to publish low quality pseudo-scientific papers. I regret not having emigrated earlier; I nearly did.

> I left rotation six months early because I realized I would be on the hospital registrars' scrap heap at the end. Increasingly no one on that rotation had achieved a senior registrar or lecturer grade in twelve years. My medical school colleagues over the country were also being shunted back into research and I'd already done twelve months' full-time research in vascular research at King's College Hospital.

> Career advancement in UK is not decided solely on merit but on many other factors. Nepotism and racism are inherent in selection process. From a surgical point of view it is distressing to see academic excellence being more important than manual ability. (Cardiothoracic surgeon in South Africa, the country of his birth)

Domestic reasons are often the cause of *return from abroad*: 'responsibility for parents', 'wife wants to return', 'children's education'.

> I will practise in UK for next twenty years as I have two children, the younger aged 4, and then return to community health in the Developing World. (Doctor who had worked in Bangladesh, Thailand and Ghana)

> I was seconded to McMaster during my training in London and might well have stayed had my visa worked out but Ontario required three years working in the frozen north first, which was not acceptable. I was recently invited to a $190,000 post in Toronto but turned it down because the upheaval too great for family.

> We had a marvellous time in Papua New Guinea but felt we should return for the benefit of the children and the longer we stayed the more difficult it would be to get back into English medicine.

This regret was echoed by another doctor working in the Third World:

> Everyone should do it, but most are scared about problems of re-entry to career in UK: should be made *less* difficult!

One doctor who found no difficulty stepping on and off the ladder went to Australia in 1976 with a view to permanent emigration, worked as a GP and started training in surgery; he returned home for family reasons and trained as a registrar in Edinburgh, and became a senior registrar in London, during which time he spent a year in Canada. At his latest reply he was an ENT surgeon in the UK.

Another respondent returned from the Karolinska Institute in Stockholm for domestic reasons, but 'if we had known about the difficulties facing developments in immunology consequent upon academic and NHS cuts since 1979 we would not have returned'. These sentiments were endorsed by one doctor, who wrote:

> Christ knows why we returned; if things do not improve in the NHS I will seriously consider emigrating to a professional academic post in the States.

These negative viewpoints tend to make the grass seem greener on the other side of the Atlantic, from either shore; one reads such remarks as 'I have a distaste for the children to be brought up as Canadians or Americans'.

More *positive reasons* are being a national of the country to which one is returning, or enjoying the country and the work. It is interesting that, in a cohort of 2,272, the number born abroad was 248 (10.9 per cent of the total). Of the 278 abroad at the time of their last reply, 59 had been born abroad (21.2 per cent). Some moved on to the USA, for example, and some returned to their homeland and took their spouse:

> I am a paediatrician in a government mission hospital in Nigeria (my husband's country); this suits me best in the present system of Nigerian medical practice and bearing in mind that I am working in a culture and language different from my own.

A similar reason is marrying a national of the country visited:

> I came to USA in 1977 on vacation, met and married an American (now a consultant chest physician); we are very fortunate that my parents are retired and come over and look after us four months every year.

This doctor enjoyed the flexibility of opportunity:

> I trained in genetics but became bored with basic research and frustrated by clinical genetics so turned to cardiology — this course would not have been a practical alternative if I had stayed in the UK.

Satisfaction with the country of emigration is a very positive reason.

> New Zealand is a beautiful and relatively unpolluted and unpopulated country.

> I came to Victoria, Australia, on a working holiday. I found it very appealing so I stayed. (Now a rural GP)

> I found flexibility available in my chosen career and a greater choice of practice venue and ability to move if desired to fit in with career and other aspirations.

> I went to Houston as a visiting professor for one year and stayed because I enjoy the life-style and working conditions.

> In just fifteen months in Canada I've paid my mortgage on a house in the UK and Canada. We own two cars and a light aircraft. We can afford two holidays a year now. Work here is enjoyable and stimulating. How could I at the age of 32 years have achieved that, even after a further ten years in the NHS? Will not return, life's too good here!

Another doctor, who emigrated to New Zealand in 1976 and was a consultant in internal medicine, spent five years as Medical Superintendent in the Solomon Islands based on Munda.

> I had a single doctored forty-six bedded general hospital serving half the Province's 50,000 coastal dwelling Melanesians, and quarterly ten-day canoe tours of all villages within 100 kilometre radius.

A woman doctor, an assistant professor in the University Family Practice Department, enjoyed the work also:

> My academic career progress is considerably better in Canada. I have more flexibility and can follow my own research pursuits in a way that would have been impossible by UK standards due to the rigidity of the NHS system.

Another respondent, content with work opportunities, wrote:

> I have an excellent job in Australia, five sessions in anaesthesia and two in intensive care, plus a session teaching computing as a lecturer at Queensland's Institute of Technology and ten lectures per year to the medical students at the University.

A consultant psychiatrist in Sydney said simply:

> Private practice offers greater flexibility and control over one's work standards.

Dissatisfaction with the new country is another reason for return.

> The advantage of the USA over the UK professionally is the freedom of work-style; the disadvantage is that it is uncivilized.

> I was disillusioned about the future prospects of a career in a private health service in an overdoctored society. (Respondent who emigrated to Australia and returned to be a GP in Suffolk)

> After specialist psychiatry training in Australia career prospects in UK improved, work-style is comparable, life-style, living conditions and financial prospects seemed less relevant than taking up the challenge of psychiatry in the UK. The travel/adventure factor diminished and I had a sense of vocation to return home near my family.

The *value of time spent abroad* is recognized by many; for one respondent:

> Two years in the Department of Thoracic Medicine in the Royal Children's Hospital, Melbourne, was the most useful job I've done. It resulted in my gaining a consultant post after only twelve months as senior registrar in UK because the quality of training in Australia is recognized to be so high.

And for others:

> I have just returned from four months in Indonesian New Guinea where I led a medical research project (with special interest in an epidemic of cysticerosis) and have made a film for a BBC-TV *World About Us* programme.

Although most permanent emigrants go to one country only, many move two or three times within it before finally settling, perhaps because mobility often leads to higher status and income, and a better climate. Thus, in reverse to UK practice, training is accomplished in one place but more movement occurs within the country later on. Often, secondment to a fellowship in the USA or elsewhere, as part of a training programme or self-arranged, gives an advantage in gaining a senior position on return; but it is likely that these doctors form an elite who would have succeeded anyway. The period spent abroad is relatively short and premeditated.

Those going for travel and adventure, and to explore a new world, often have no time limit or definite end in view, and their future career depends on what they find in the unknown. But some go to take an exploratory look first, or return to compare conditions in this country before a define decision to emigrate is finally made. Some find their decision made for them by domestic circumstances — the preference of a spouse, the education of children, or the welfare of parents. Those engaged in missionary work and Third World medicine are sometimes on short-term contracts but more often have a long-term commitment. They include those for whom Third World medicine means research in centres of excellence rather than fieldwork.

Emigration is a many faceted subject. It is of value to those doctors who go for self-development, and to the host countries, who gain by cross-fertilization of medical ideas. It is sad that emigration should be inhibited by national fears of doctor overproduction, rigid career structures, and the anxieties of trainees, since global movement of doctors, like all international cooperation, is of great benefit to us all.

THE 1977, 1980 AND 1983 QUALIFIERS

We looked at the position of these doctors, with regard to international movement, at comparable periods of time — in April of alternate years after qualifying. For 1983 qualifiers this gave information about where respondents were, and what they were doing three years after qualifying — in April 1986. For 1980 qualifiers it gave information for three and five years after qualifying, and for 1977 qualifiers, for three, five and nine years after qualifying. In real time, therefore, the information relating to 1983 qualifiers after three years, and to 1977 qualifiers after nine years, refers in both cases to what was happening to them in April 1986.

Table 7.8 shows the proportions of male and female respondents who were known to be abroad at the times concerned. Three years after qualifying, slightly higher proportions of men than women were abroad in all three cohorts; but five years after qualifying this situation was reversed and after nine years the proportions of men and women abroad were almost equal. Altogether, higher proportions of respondents were abroad at the five-year point than at the three-year point, and the highest proportion was for 1977 qualifiers nine years after leaving medical school. At both three years and five years after qualifying, higher proportions of 1977 qualifiers than 1980 qualifiers were abroad, and the lowest proportion was among 1983 qualifiers at their three year point.

Table 7.8 Percentages of respondents abroad at April of year shown

Year of qualifying		*Years after qualifying*		
		3 years	*5 years*	*9 years*
1983	Men	3.6		
	Women	3.0		
	Total	3.3		
1980	Men	4.3	5.7	
	Women	4.1	6.1	
	Total	4.2	5.8	
1977	Men	7.1	8.4	10.0
	Women	6.9	9.4	10.1
	Total	7.1	8.7	10.0

Table 7.9 Percentages of respondents having been abroad by April of year shown

Year of qualifying		*Years after qualifying*		
		3 years	*5 years*	*9 years*
1983	Men	6.2		
	Women	5.6		
	Total	6.0		
1980	Men	8.0	12.5	
	Women	6.2	12.4	
	Total	7.4	12.5	
1977	Men	9.2	15.8	25.3
	Women	8.5	15.5	23.1
	Total	9.0	15.7	24.6

Table 7.8 refers to the respondents who were actually abroad in April of the years concerned. Table 7.9 gives a cumulative picture of the numbers of respondents who had been abroad, including those still abroad, by the lengths of time shown after

Table 7.10 Intentions of practising in UK (percentages of those known to have been abroad at some time)

Year of qualifying		*Years after qualifying*		
		3 years	*5 years*	*9 years*
1983	Definitely yes	22.6		
	Definitely no	9.3		
	Probably yes	36.3		
	Probably no	13.3		
	Undecided	18.5		
1980	Definitely yes	28.2	30.5	
	Definitely no	5.3	7.4	
	Probably yes	40.2	34.4	
	Probably no	11.1	10.9	
	Undecided	15.2	16.9	
1977	Definitely yes	22.4	26.2	33.7
	Definitely no	3.1	7.2	11.6
	Probably yes	34.5	34.1	26.0
	Probably no	6.4	11.0	11.5
	Undecided	33.6	21.4	17.1

leaving medical school. The general picture amplifies the conclusions of Table 7.8, and gives confirmation to the evidence offered in other chapters that movement abroad diminished for the successive cohorts in our studies. Three years after leaving medical school, 9.0 per cent of 1977 qualifiers had been abroad and 7.1 per cent were actually abroad, compared to 6.0 per cent of 1983 qualifiers who had been abroad and only 3.3 per cent who were actually abroad at the time. By nine years after qualifying, almost 25 per cent of 1977 qualifiers had been abroad at some stage.

Table 7.10 shows the intentions of respondents about whether they would ultimately plan to practise in the UK. The figures are percentages of those qualifiers know to have been abroad at some time. Among these doctors, the proportions who definitely intended to practise in the UK, and also the proportions of those who definitely intended not to practise in the UK, rose steadily as the years passed after leaving medical school. Nine years after qualifying, 11.6 per cent of 1977 qualifiers who had been abroad

Table 7.11 Countries of respondents (percentages of those abroad at times shown)

Countries	Year of qualifying	Years after qualifying: 3 years	5 years	9 years
Europe	1983	25.2		
	1980	17.1	14.5	
	1977	11.4	15.4	9.0
Australia	1983	14.8		
	1980	7.4	14.5	
	1977	12.8	10.8	17.3
New Zealand	1983	6.1		
	1980	7.4	10.8	
	1977	17.6	11.5	8.3
Canada	1983	5.2		
	1980	11.9	13.4	
	1977	10.0	15.0	16.0
USA	1983	13.0		
	1980	8.9	12.4	
	1977	9.5	10.8	14.0
Other	1983	35.7		
	1980	47.4	34.4	
	1977	38.9	36.6	35.3

indicated that they definitely did not intend to return to the UK. Correspondingly the proportions of respondents who were undecided about their future plans not surprisingly declined as they went further into their postgraduate careers.

Table 7.11 shows the countries in which respondents were working in April of the years concerned. The figures are percentages of respondents who were known to be abroad at the times shown. Three years after qualifying, the proportions of respondents in Europe were greater among 1980 qualifiers than 1977 qualifiers, and greater again, by a considerable degree, among 1983 qualifiers. In all cases the great majority of these doctors were working in EC countries. Over 25 per cent of the 1983 qualifiers who were abroad in April 1986 were in Europe; at the same date, only 9.0 per cent of the 1977 qualifiers who were abroad at that time were in Europe. Australia was a much

Table 7.12 Specialties of respondents (percentages of those abroad at times shown)

	Years after qualifying and year of qualifying					
	3 years			*5 years*		*9 years*
Specialty	*1977*	*1980*	*1983*	*1977*	*1980*	*1977*
Medicine	25.1	20.7	20.9	17.7	16.7	14.3
Surgery	11.8	5.2	7.8	10.0	7.0	12.3
Obstetrics and gynaecology	3.8	4.4	4.3	1.9	5.9	2.7
Anaesthetics	5.2	2.2	0.9	7.3	3.2	9.7
Pathology	0.5	0.7	2.6	1.5	2.2	1.3
Psychiatry	1.9	4.4	2.6	1.9	4.8	2.7
Radiology/radiotherapy	1.9	–	2.6	3.5	1.1	3.3
Community medicine	0.5	0.7	0.9	1.5	1.1	1.3
General practice	24.6	25.2	29.6	28.1	29.6	30.3
Third World medicine	11.8	6.7	6.1	8.8	9.1	10.0
Other/none	12.8	29.6	21.7	17.7	19.4	12.0

less popular venue, three years after qualifying, among 1980 qualifiers than for the other two cohorts, and New Zealand was outstandingly popular among 1977 qualifiers. The proportions of respondents working in Canada and the USA rose steadily as the years went by from leaving medical school. Relatively more of the recent qualifiers, however, were in the USA than in Canada: in April 1986, forty-two 1977 respondents and fifteen 1983 respondents were in the USA (14 and 13 per cent of the numbers abroad), while in Canada there were forty-eight 1977 respondents and only six 1983 respondents (16 and 5.2 per cent of those abroad).

Table 7.12 shows the type of work being done by respondents who were abroad three, five and nine years after qualifying. General practice, either alone or combined with hospital work, was the most popular option throughout. The lowest proportion of respondents engaged in Third World medicine was among 1983 qualifiers three years after leaving medical school. However, at this stage of their careers only a slightly higher proportion of 1980 qualifiers were engaged in this kind of work, but the proportion had risen to over 9.0 per cent two years later. About 10.0 per cent of the 1977 qualifiers who were abroad at any of the three times studied were doing this kind of work. Among the hospital specialties, medicine was the most popular option for work abroad, but more in the early years after qualifying than later. Conversely the proportions of 1977 respondents who were working abroad in anaesthetics and radiology/radiotherapy were higher five and nine years after qualifying than three years after qualifying.

It is difficult to make direct comparisons between the three cohorts regarding the lengths of time spent abroad, since the 1983 qualifiers were followed for only three years. Among the 1977 qualifiers, followed for nine years, about 25 per cent of those who had been abroad had spent more than four years out of the UK. For all three cohorts, the commonest total length of time to be spent abroad was either six to twelve months or one to two years. Among the respondents who had been abroad, 40 per cent of 1977 qualifiers, 45.5 per cent of 1980s and 59.2 per cent of 1983s had spent altogether between six months and two years abroad.

Of the 1977 respondents who were known to have been abroad at some time, 61.8 per cent were known to be back in the UK when they last replied to us; this compared to 59.8 per cent of the corresponding 1980 qualifiers, and 47.8 per cent of those who qualified in 1983 and were known to have been abroad. The decline in the total amount of international movement over the years studied is illustrated by the fact that, although the total number of 1977 qualifiers was the smallest of the three years here considered, and although the percentage known to be back in the UK from abroad was the highest for the three cohorts, the absolute number of doctors who qualified in 1977 and were estimated to be still abroad at their latest reply to us was 285, compared to 174 who qualified in 1980 and 118 who qualified in 1983.

8 Career progress

Employment status of doctors

For medical personnel planning it is of great importance to estimate the working capacity, and also the actual work contribution, of a given set of doctors. We have used our data for such studies, and this chapter reports on the employment status of two of our cohorts at comparable periods after qualifying — the 1974 qualifiers in 1979, and the 1977 qualifiers in 1982.

THE 1974 QUALIFIERS IN 1979

The employment status of these doctors was taken to be their occupation in or around November 1979 (Parkhouse *et al.* 1982). This was when our 1979 questionnaires were first sent out. These questionnaires gave us the employment status of 74.9 per cent of the doctors known to have qualified in the calendar year 1974. A total of 269 doctors who were non-respondents in 1979 replied in 1981, giving details of the posts they had held in 1979. The DHSS then supplied aggregate details for a further 191 qualifiers out of 250 whom we believed to have been practising in the UK in 1979. Later, we received questionnaire replies which gave information for a further seven doctors. Altogether, from these sources, we compiled information about 94.9 per cent of the 1974 qualifiers. Of the 120 who remained untraced, 39 were thought to be in the UK at the time of the 1979 survey, and all these had addresses in the principal list of the 1979 Medical Register. Seventy-one others were not in the Register, and could not have been practising medicine legitimately in the UK; the last known addresses of fifty-four of them were abroad. A further ten, though on the Register, were also thought to be overseas from their last known addresses. There remained, therefore, only seventeen qualifiers (0.7 per cent) whose location and occupation were unknown. None of these was in the 1979 Medical Register.

Table 8.1 Employment status in 1979, by sex (1974 qualifiers)[a]

Occupation group	Men		Women		Unknown		Total	
United Kingdom								
NHS[b]	1,296	(75.8)	444	(70.7)	0		1,740	(74.0)
Universities	43	(2.5)	7	(1.1)	0		50	(2.1)
Other public sector	43	(2.5)	12	(1.9)	0		55	(2.3)
Public sector total	1,382	(80.3)	463	(73.7)	0		1,845	(78.5)
Non-public sector	6	(0.3)	3	(0.5)	0		9	(0.4)
Non-medical	5	(0.3)	0		0		5	(0.2)
Unemployed	22	(1.3)	89	(14.2)	0		111	(4.7)
Unknown but in 1979 Medical Register	23	(1.3)	16	(2.5)	0		39	(1.7)
UK total	1,438	(83.6)	571	(90.9)	0		2,009	(85.4)
Armed Forces	54	(3.1)	1	(0.2)	0		55	(2.3)
Abroad								
Medical	154	(9.0)	36	(5.7)	0		190	(8.1)
Unemployed	3	(0.2)	8	(1.3)	0		11	(0.5)
Unknown	53	(3.1)	10	(1.6)	1	(50)	64	(2.7)
Abroad total	210	(12.2)	54	(8.6)	1	(50)	265	(11.2)
Deceased	4	(0.2)	0		0		4	(0.2)
Unknown	14	(0.8)	2	(0.3)	1	(50)	17	(0.7)
Total	1,720	(100)	628	(100)	2	(100)	2,350	(100)

Notes: a Figures shown are total numbers with percentages in parentheses
b Includes fifteen men and four women apparently in partly NHS and partly university or other public sector posts

Source: Reproduced by permission from the *BMJ*, Parkhouse *et al.* 1982

Employment status

We assigned doctors to occupation groups on the basis of the rules and occupation groups used by the DHSS. Each doctor was counted once only, priority being given to the more 'important' post, that is, the post appearing nearest the top of the DHSS list. On this basis, doctors holding university posts together with honorary NHS appointments were assigned to the university group, except that holders of research registrar and research senior registrar posts were counted as NHS. The category 'other public sector' included doctors employed by the Medical Research Council, the Public Health Laboratory Services, the Department of Employment, and the DHSS. 'Non-public sector' included doctors employed by industrial organizations, and those in private practice.

Fifteen men and four women appeared to be employed partly in the NHS and partly in other appointments. They were included in the total of doctors working for the NHS. Table 8.1 gives a general breakdown of employment status, and Table 8.2 analyses the employment status of those doctors who were working in the NHS.

There were 1,296 men (75.3 per cent) and 444 women (70.7 per cent) known to be working for the NHS five years after qualifying, a total of 1,740 doctors (74 per cent). For the whole of the public sector — i.e. the NHS plus the universities, the MRC and other public sector employees — the numbers working were 1,382 men (80.3 per cent) and 463 women (73.7 per cent), a total of 1,845 (78.5 per cent).

It is difficult to obtain accurate information about doctors known to be working outside the public sector, to have left medicine, or to have died. These numbers were small, but the figures quoted in Table 8.1 may be underestimates. The twenty-three men and sixteen women who were not definitely traced but whose names were in the 1979 Medical Register were probably practising in the UK; some of these could have been working outside the public sector. Thus, a total of 1,411 men (82 per cent) and 482 women (76.8 per cent) were known or thought to be practising medicine in the UK — an overall rate of 80.6 per cent.

In 1979 265 doctors (11.3 per cent) were known or presumed from their last known addresses to be living abroad. The true number may be slightly higher, since a majority of the seventeen qualifiers with unknown occupation and location may well have been abroad.

Table 8.2 NHS employment status in 1979, by sex (1974 qualifiers)[a]

Grade	*Men*		*Women*		*Total*	
Hospital						
Senior hospital doctor						
Consultant[b]	2	(0.1)	1	(0.2)	3	(0.1)
Senior registrar	123	(7.2)	25	(4.0)	148	(6.3)
Other	2	(0.1)	1	(0.2)	3	(0.1)
Total	127	(7.4)	27	(4.3)	154	(6.6)
Junior hospital doctor						
Registrar	476	(27.7)	119	(18.9)	595	(25.3)
SHO	117	(6.8)	43	(6.8)	160	(6.8)
House officer	0		2	(0.3)	2	(0.1)
Other	6	(0.3)	0		6	(0.3)
Total	599	(34.8)	164	(26.1)	763	(32.5)
Part-time hospital medical officer	4	(0.2)	12	(1.9)	16	(0.7)
Hospital total	730	(42.4)	203	(32.3)	933	(39.7)
Non-hospital						
General practitioner	552	(32.1)	202	(32.2)	754	(32.1)
Post in community health service[c]	14	(0.8)	39	(6.2)	53	(2.3)
Non-hospital total	566	(32.9)	241	(38.4)	807	(34.3)
Total	1,296	(75.3)	444	(70.7)	1,740	(74.0)

Notes: a Figures shown are total numbers, with percentages in parentheses
b Includes one man and one woman with locum appointments, and one man with previous dental training who was a consultant in oral surgery. In addition, one man employed as a consultant in oral medicine in the Army also had previous dental training
c Includes one man in ophthalmic medical practice

Source: Reproduced by permission from the *BMJ*, Parkhouse *et al.* 1982

Part-time employment

There were 150 women working part-time in the NHS (33.7 per cent of women known to be working for the NHS). The number of sessions worked ranged from less than one to nine, and was unknown in seven cases. The commonest numbers of sessions worked were five, six and two (twenty-seven, twenty-five and twenty-three doctors respectively). The mean number of weekly sessions was 4.5. There were ten men for whom a part-time NHS post was the only known employment. One was working five sessions a week, but the numbers of sessions worked by the nine others, only one of whom had replied to the questionnaires, were unknown.

A further fifteen men and four women appeared, from their responses, to be working part-time for the NHS while holding other appointments, usually academic or research posts. The actual numbers of sessions worked by all but one of these doctors were unknown.

Whole-time equivalents

The actual work contribution of doctors is not accurately described by counting the numbers of doctors who are employed, because of the fact that some work only part-time. Table 8.3 shows the estimated whole-time equivalent work contribution of 1974 qualifiers in 1979. In this table, doctors who were working purely part-time, for an unknown number of sessions, were assumed to be working five NHS sessions a week. The nineteen doctors who appeared to be working partly for the NHS and partly for other public sector employers were assumed to be working five NHS and five non-NHS sessions a week. The work contribution of untraced qualifiers was estimated as described in the footnotes to the table.

From our study, the overall contribution of 1974 qualifiers to the NHS agreed with recent projections that of all British-born civilian doctors *in Great Britain*, a percentage whole-time equivalent of 80-85 per cent were working in the NHS. However, allowing for doctors working in the Armed Forces or overseas, the true whole-time equivalent contribution to the NHS for all qualifiers was only 69.9 per cent (excluding those in universities with honorary NHS contracts). For the public sector in general — NHS, universities, MRC, etc. — the whole-time equivalent contribution for all qualifiers was 74.7 per cent. Their overall contribution to medicine, including non-public sector work, the Armed Forces, and work abroad, was 90.1 per cent.

Table 8.3 Estimated whole-time equivalent posts in medicine, by sex (1974 qualifiers)[a]

Occupation group	*Men*		*Women*		*Unknown*		*Total*	
United Kingdom								
NHS	1,283.2	(74.6)	360.5	(57.4)	0		1,643.7	(69.9)
Universities	46.0	(2.7)	6.5	(1.0)	0		52.5	(2.2)
Other public sector	46.8	(2.7)	13.0	(2.1)	0		59.8	(2.5)
Public sector total	1,376.0	(80.0)	380.0	(60.5)	0		1,756.0	(74.7)
Non-public sector	6.0	(0.3)	1.2	(0.2)	0		7.2	(0.3)
Unknown but in 1979 Medical Register[b]	22.5	(1.3)	11.0	(1.8)	0		33.5	(1.4)
UK total	1,404.5	(81.7)	392.2	(62.5)	0		1,796.6	(76.5)
Armed Forces	54.0	(3.1)	1.0	(0.2)	0		55.0	(2.3)
Abroad								
Medical	154.0	(9.0)	35.1	(5.6)	0		189.1	(8.0)
Unknown[c]	52.0	(3.0)	8.0	(1.3)	1	(50)	61.0	(2.6)
Abroad total	206.0	(12.0)	43.1	(6.9)	1	(50)	250.1	(10.6)
Unknown[d]	13.7	(0.8)	1.4	(0.2)	1	(50)	16.1	(0.7)
Total	1,678.2	(97.6)	437.7	(69.7)	2	(100)	2,117.9	(90.1)

Notes: a Figures shown are total numbers, with percentages in parentheses
b Twenty-three men and sixteen women; wte contributions estimated proportionately using all other UK figures
c Fifty-three men, ten women and one of unknown sex; wte contributions estimated proportionately using all other abroad figures
d Fourteen men, two women and one of unknown sex; wte contributions estimated proportionately using all other figures

Source: Reproduced by permission from the *BMJ*, Parkhouse *et al.* 1982

Medical school differences

The percentage of 1974 qualifiers still working for the NHS five years after qualifying varied from 60.4 per cent for Oxford graduates to 84.9 per cent for those from the University of Wales College of Medicine. St Bartholomew's Hospital showed the highest proportion of qualifiers employed in universities (6.0 per cent), while most of Oxford's 6.3 per cent who were working for other public sector employers were with the MRC. The total percentages of qualifiers working in the public sector ranged from 70.8 per cent for Oxford to 87.1 per cent for St George's Hospital. There were slightly higher percentages of qualifiers working in the NHS or other public sector posts from provincial medical schools in England than from London medical schools, but the corresponding overall percentages for Scottish medical schools were rather lower.

Of qualifiers from the Royal Free Hospital, 13.2 per cent were in the UK but not in regular employment — by far the largest proportion of unemployed qualifiers for medical schools in England and Wales. However, 48.4 per cent of the Royal Free Hospital qualifiers were women, and ten of these forty-four were unemployed. Unemployment in the UK was also high for Aberdeen (9.5 per cent of all qualifiers) and Dundee (10.6 per cent) mainly because of nine and seven women respectively from these medical schools who were not working. This raised the combined rate for Scottish medical schools to 6.0 per cent, considerably above the overall figure of 4.7 per cent.

Among qualifiers abroad, fourteen were from Sheffield (17.5 per cent) and thirty-three from Glasgow (17.4 per cent), compared to only three from Charing Cross Hospital (7.5 per cent). Overall, the emigration rate was highest for Scottish medical school qualifiers, and slightly higher for London qualifiers than for English provincial medical school qualifiers.

The medical schools in Northern England — Leeds, Liverpool, Manchester, Newcastle and Sheffield — and in Glasgow showed higher percentages of qualifiers in general practice than in the hospital service. Overall, there were slightly more qualifiers from the provincial medical schools in general practice than in hospital posts; but the reverse was true for qualifiers from London medical schools, the University of Wales College of Medicine, and Scottish medical schools.

The percentage of qualifiers in community medicine and community health was highest from Charing Cross Hospital (7.5 per cent) and Manchester (5.5 per cent), though this represented only three and eight doctors respectively.

Unemployment

In the UK twenty-two men (1.3 per cent) and eighty-nine women (14.2 per cent) were not in regular employment at the time of the 1979 survey — a total of 111 qualifiers (4.7 per cent). Of these, four men and five women were doing occasional work of some kind.

Most unemployed women were temporarily out of medical practice for domestic reasons. From questionnaire replies it seemed that several other doctors were temporarily unavailable for employment, for example because they were studying for examinations or moving. At least four men and three women were waiting to take up their next post. Allowing for such qualifiers, there seemed to be at most thirteen men (0.8 per cent of all men and 0.9 per cent of those known or thought to be in the UK) and thirty women (4.8 per cent of all women and 5.3 per cent of those in the UK) who were available for work but could not find suitable employment. This combined total of forty-three represented 1.8 per cent of all qualifiers and 2.1 per cent of those known or thought to be in the UK. Unemployment therefore did not seem to be a serious problem, but it was noticeable that some women anticipated, or had actually experienced, difficulty in finding employment of a kind compatible with their domestic arrangements.

THE 1977 QUALIFIERS IN 1982

The latest three questionnaire replies from 1977 qualifiers provided most of the data for this study (Ellin and Parkhouse 1989). From questionnaire returns we were able to discover the employment status of 87.7 per cent of 3,136 qualifiers in the calendar year 1977. The DHSS provided aggregate employment information for a further 300 doctors (9.6 per cent) for their annual census date of 30 September 1982. Eight doctors had died before November 1982, so that altogether we had job data for 3,059 doctors (97.5 per cent). Of the remaining seventy-seven doctors, thirty-six were in the Medical Register for 1982 and had addresses in the UK. A further eleven were registered, but thought to be abroad. Nineteen doctors not in the 1982 Medical Register were thought from their latest addresses and responses to be abroad. There remained, therefore, eleven doctors, not on the Register, whose location was unknown (0.35 per cent).

Employment status

This study included qualifiers from the newly developed clinical school at Cambridge; from Queen's University, Belfast, which was not included in the 1974 cohort; and from the new medical schools of Southampton and Nottingham, which were not producing graduates in 1974. Figures are calculated using information from all these medical schools, but Tables 8.4 and 8.5 also show results calculated only for the medical schools which were included in the survey of 1974 qualifiers in 1979.

Doctors holding two or more jobs of different kinds concurrently were assigned to a single occupation, again using DHSS rules of precedence. This applied to seventy-nine doctors (2.5 per cent); 44 per cent of these were working mainly in general practice full-time or nearly full-time, and a further fifteen (all women) were part-time general practitioners with other work as well. In this survey, thirty research registrars and one research senior registrar were included in the university sector, rather than the NHS.

The improved proportion of traced qualifiers (97.5 per cent compared to 94.9 per cent in the earlier study) increases the numbers in some of the occupational groups in the UK to a few tenths of a percentage point above the level that would have resulted from identical detection rates in the two studies. The main difference is a much lower number of doctors of unknown occupation presumed to be abroad; bearing this in mind, background calculations show that the slight distorting factor of a higher detection rate had a negligible influence, so that for the two studies as a whole, grounds for comparison remain very sound.

Table 8.4 shows that, compared to 1974 qualifiers in 1979, there was a notable increase from 85.4 to 88.0 per cent in the proportion of doctors resident in the UK. This was a major reason for the marked expansion of all medical occupation groups in the UK for men and women combined. For example the percentage of doctors working for the NHS had risen quite sharply from 74.0 to 77.1 per cent, and for the public sector as a whole there was a 4.1 percentage point increase to 82.6 per cent of qualifiers.

Table 8.5 gives a breakdown of the employment status of the 2,418 doctors working in the NHS. In general practice and community medicine, apart from marginal expansion of the latter, the proportions of qualifiers had remained virtually the same as for 1974 qualifiers in 1979. In hospital medicine, 34.7 per cent of qualifiers held posts, compared to 32.5 per cent of

Table 8.4 Employment status five years after qualifying, by sex (1977 qualifiers)[a]

	Men				Women				Total			
Occupation group	*All 1977s*		*1974s*	*'Old'[b] 1977s*	*All 1977s*		*1974s*	*'Old'[b] 1977s*	*All 1977s*		*1974s*	*'Old'[b] 1977s*
United Kingdom												
NHS[c]	1,658	(78.3)	(75.3)[d]	(79.0)	760	(74.6)	(70.7)	(75.2)	2,418	(77.1)	(74.0)	(77.8)
Universities	56	(2.6)	(2.5)	(2.7)	12	(1.2)	(1.1)	(1.2)	68	(2.2)	(2.1)	(2.2)
Other public sector	82	(3.9)	(2.5)	(3.7)	23	(2.3)	(1.9)	(2.2)	105	(3.3)	(2.3)	(3.2)
Public sector total	1,796	(84.8)	(80.3)	(85.4)	795	(78.0)	(73.7)	(78.6)	2,591	(82.6)	(78.5)	(83.2)
Non-public sector	16	(0.8)	(0.3)	(0.8)	3	(0.3)	(0.5)	(0.3)	19	(0.6)	(0.4)	(0.6)
Non-medical	1	–	(0.3)	–	2	(0.2)	0.0	(0.2)	3	(0.1)	(0.2)	(0.1)
Unemployed	20	(0.9)	(1.3)	(1.0)	91	(8.9)	(14.2)	(8.9)	111	(3.5)	(4.7)	(3.5)
Unknown but in 1982 Medical Register	21	(1.0)	(1.3)	(0.8)	15	(1.5)	(2.5)	(1.0)	36	(1.1)	(1.7)	(0.9)
UK total	1,854	(87.6)	(83.6)	(88.0)	906	(88.9)	(90.9)	(89.0)	2,760	(88.0)	(85.4)	(88.3)
Armed Forces	71	(3.4)	(3.1)	(3.3)	6	(0.6)	(0.2)	(0.5)	77	(2.5)	(2.3)	(2.4)
Abroad												
Medical	149	(7.0)	(9.0)	(6.8)	70	(6.9)	(5.7)	(6.7)	219	(7.0)	(8.1)	(6.7)
Non-medical	2	(0.1)	0.0	(0.1)	1	(0.1)	0.0	(0.1)	3	(0.1)	0.0	(0.1)
Unemployed	7	(0.3)	(0.2)	(0.4)	21	(2.1)	(1.3)	(2.0)	28	(0.9)	(0.5)	(0.9)
Unknown	23	(1.1)	(3.1)	(1.0)	7	(0.7)	(1.6)	(0.8)	30	(1.0)	(2.7)	(0.9)
Abroad total	181	(8.5)	(12.2)	(8.2)	99	(9.7)	(8.6)	(9.6)	280	(8.9)	(11.2)	(8.7)

Table 8.4 continued

Occupation group	*Men*			*Women*			*Total*		
	All 1977s	*1974s*	*'Old'*[b] *1977s*	*All 1977s*	*1974s*	*'Old'*[b] *1977s*	*All 1977s*	*1974s*	*'Old'*[b] *1977s*
Deceased	6 (0.3)	(0.2)	(0.3)	2 (0.2)	0.0	(0.2)	8 (0.3)	(0.2)	(0.3)
Unknown	5 (0.2)	(0.8)	(0.2)	6 (0.6)	(0.3)	(0.7)	11 (0.4)	(0.7)	(0.3)
Total	2,117 (100.0)	(100.0)	(100.0)	1,019 (100.0)	(100.0)	(100.0)	3,136 (100.0)	(100.0)	(100.0)

Notes: a Figures shown are total numbers, with percentages in parentheses

b 'Old' medical schools indicate schools surveyed in 1979 study (i.e. excluding Belfast, Cambridge, Nottingham and Southampton); total for 1979 study includes two doctors of unknown sex

c Includes thirteen people working partly in the NHS in 1982 and partly in: universities (one man); other public sector (two men, one woman); non-public sector (five men, four women). In Table 8.6 the sessions worked by these people have been apportioned between the relevant sectors: a similar adjustment was made to the 1979 study

d Wrongly shown as 75.8 in the 1979 study

Percentages that are less than 0.1 are shown as a dash

Table 8.5 NHS employment status five years after qualifying, by sex (1977 qualifiers)[a]

	Men				Women				Total			
Occupation group	*All 1977s*		*1974s*	*'Old'[b] 1977s*	*All 1977s*		*1974s*	*'Old'[b] 1977s*	*All 1977s*		*1974s*	*'Old'[b] 1977s*
Hospital												
Senior hospital doctor												
Consultant[c]	1	0.0	(0.1)	(0.1)	2	(0.2)	(0.2)	(0.2)	3	(0.1)	(0.1)	(0.1)
Senior registrar	136	(6.4)	(7.2)	(5.9)	59	(5.8)	(4.0)	(5.5)	195	(6.2)	(6.3)	(5.8)
Other	0	0.0	(0.1)	0.0	1	(0.1)	(0.2)	(0.1)	1	–	(0.1)	–
Total	137	(6.5)	(7.4)	(6.0)	62	(6.1)	(4.3)	(5.9)	199	(6.3)	(6.6)	(6.0)
Junior hospital doctor												
Registrar	637	(30.1)	(27.7)	(30.4)	199	(19.5)	(18.9)	(19.6)	836	(26.7)	(25.3)	(27.0)
SHO	172	(8.1)	(6.8)	(8.4)	72	(7.1)	(6.8)	(7.0)	244	(7.8)	(6.8)	(8.0)
House Officer	1	–	0.0	–	0.0	0.0	(0.3)	0.0	1	–	(0.1)	–
Other	3	(0.1)	(0.3)	(0.2)	5	(0.5)	0.0	(0.5)	8	(0.3)	(0.3)	(0.3)
Total	813	(38.4)	(34.8)	(39.1)	276	(27.1)	(26.1)	(27.1)	1,089	(34.7)	(32.5)	(35.2)
Part-time hospital MO	10	(0.5)	(0.2)	(0.5)	23	(2.3)	(1.9)	(2.4)	33	(1.1)	(0.7)	(1.1)
Hospital total	960	(45.3)	(42.4)	(45.6)	361	(35.4)	(32.3)	(35.3)	1,321	(42.1)	(39.7)	(42.3)

Table 8.5 continued

Occupation group	Men			Women			Total		
	All 1977s	*1974s*	*'Old'[b] 1977s*	*All 1977s*	*1974s*	*'Old'[b] 1977s*	*All 1977s*	*1974s*	*'Old'[b] 1977s*
Non-hospital									
General practitioner	680 (32.1)	(32.1)	(32.6)	327 (32.1)	(32.2)	(32.7)	1,007 (32.1)	(32.1)	(32.6)
Post in community medicine[d]	18[e] (0.9)	(0.8)	(0.8)	72 (7.1)	(6.2)	(7.2)	90 (2.9)	(2.3)	(2.8)
Non-hospital total	698 (33.0)	(32.9)	(33.4)	399 (39.2)	(38.4)	(39.9)	1,097 (35.0)	(34.3)	(35.5)
Total	1,658 (78.3)	(75.3)	(79.0)	760 (74.6)	(70.7)	(75.2)	2,418 (77.1)	(74.0)	(77.8)

Notes: a Figures shown are total numbers, with percentages in parentheses
b 'Old' medical schools indicate schools surveyed in 1979 study (i.e. excluding Belfast, Cambridge, Nottingham and Southampton)
c Includes one woman with what is presumed to be a locum appointment in 1982 (also see 1979 study)
d Includes community health
e Includes one man in ophthalmic medical practice in 1982 (also see 1979 study)
Percentages that are less than 0.1 are shown as a dash

Table 8.6 Estimated whole-time equivalent posts held in medicine five years after qualifying, by sex (1977 qualifiers)[a]

Occupation group	Men			Women			Total		
		1977s	*1974s*		*1977s*	*1974s*		*1977s*	*1974s*
United Kingdom									
NHS	1,651.6	(78.0)	(74.6)	658.8	(64.7)	(57.4)	2,310.4	(73.7)	(69.9)
Universities	56.5	(2.7)	(2.7)	12.0	(1.2)	(1.0)	68.5	(2.2)	(2.2)
Other public sector	82.2	(3.9)	(2.7)	22.7	(2.2)	(2.1)	104.9	(3.3)	(2.5)
Public sector total	1,790.3	(84.6)	(80.0)	693.5	(68.1)	(60.5)	2,483.8	(79.2)	(74.7)
Non-public sector	18.9	(0.9)	(0.3)	4.4	(0.4)	(0.2)	23.3	(0.7)	(0.3)
Unknown but in 1982 Medical Register[b]	20.7	(1.0)	(1.3)	11.7	(1.1)	(1.8)	32.4	(1.0)	(1.4)
UK total	1,829.9	(86.4)	(81.7)	709.6	(69.6)	(62.5)	2,539.5	(81.0)	(76.5)
Armed Forces	71.0	(3.4)	(3.1)	6.0	(0.6)	(0.2)	77.0	(2.5)	(2.3)

Table 8.6 continued

Occupation group	*Men*			*Women*			*Total*		
		1977s	*1974s*		*1977s*	*1974s*		*1977s*	*1974s*
Abroad									
Medical	148.6	(7.0)	(9.0)	64.7	(6.3)	(5.6)	213.3	(6.8)	(8.0)
Unknown[c]	21.6	(1.0)	(3.0)	4.9	(0.5)	(1.3)	26.5	(0.8)	(2.6)
Abroad total	170.2	(8.0)	(12.0)	69.6	(6.8)	(6.9)	239.8	(7.6)	(10.6)
Unknown[d]	4.9	(0.2)	(0.8)	4.7	(0.5)	(0.2)	9.6	(0.3)	(0.7)
Total	2,076.0	(98.1)	(97.6)	789.9	(77.5)	(69.7)	2,865.9	(91.4)	(90.1)

Notes: a Figures shown are total numbers, with percentages in parentheses; total for 1979 study includes two doctors of unknown sex
b Twenty-one men and fifteen women in 1982; wte contributions estimated proportionately using all other UK figures
c Twenty-three men and seven women in 1982; wte contributions estimated proportionately using all other abroad figures
d Five men and six women in 1982; wte contributions estimated proportionately using all other figures; similar calculations were made for the 1979 study

the previous group. The increase in NHS-employed doctors was in the hospital service and, specifically, this expansion had occurred (in both proportional and numerical terms) among SHOs and registrars, with approximately 35 per cent of NHS-based qualifiers being in the registrar grade and 10 per cent in SHO posts at this point in their careers. This increase was consistent with the higher proportion of SHO and registrar posts occupied by British rather than overseas graduates in 1982, compared with 1979. The position in the senior registrar grade remained relatively static.

Part-time employment

Work occupying less than ten half-days a week (ten sessions) was designated as part-time. In the few cases where questionnaire replies did not specify the number of sessions, the amount of work undertaken was either estimated or shown as unknown. The DHSS provided information for eleven doctors who were working part-time, but without sessional details, and their contribution was estimated. Where two or more posts were held concurrently, the number of sessions was taken as the sum of all those worked, subject to a full-time ceiling of ten sessions.

In the NHS 186 women (24.5 per cent) were working part-time in 1982. As a proportion, this was a substantial fall from the 33.8 per cent of women qualifying in 1974 who were working part-time in 1979. Because of the increased output of the medical schools and the higher proportion of women graduates, however, the absolute number of women who were working part-time was higher in 1982. The average number of sessions (4.7) showed only a marginal rise, from 4.5 for the 1974 qualifiers.

Whole-time equivalents

Table 8.6 shows that the reduced proportion of women doctors working part-time, together with a fall in unemployment among women doctors, had raised the whole-time equivalent contribution by women to medicine in the UK, compared to the 1979 survey of 1974 qualifiers, from 62.5 to 69.6 per cent of the potential full-time contribution of all the women in the respective cohorts. This considerable change had occurred against the background of a 2.0 per cent fall in the proportion of women doctors resident in the UK, thus making the increased UK contribution all the more impressive.

The shift towards whole-time work can be demonstrated by a 'crude participation rate' (CPR), which expresses participation in medicine as the average whole-time equivalent per doctor working in any particular sector. This helps to clarify the information in Table 8.6, and links it to the numbers of doctors employed (Table 8.4). The change in CPR for NHS-employed women doctors, compared to 1974 qualifiers in 1979, was from 8.12 to 8.67 weekly sessions. For all women doctors working in the UK it rose from 8.14 to 8.73. For men and women combined, in the UK, the CPR rose from 9.49 to 9.60 — a small alteration considering the substantial change noted for women doctors. Not only is the increasing commitment of female doctors to medicine largely submerged by the weight of male numbers, but also the increased proportion of women among medical graduates has the effect of reducing the overall participation rate.

Medical school differences

NHS employment was highest among the fifty-four qualifiers from Charing Cross Hospital (85.2 per cent) and the Westminster Hospital (84.6 per cent), while the Southampton medical school gave the lowest figure (66.7 per cent). University appointments were commonest among St George's Hospital qualifiers; Oxford, as noted for 1974 qualifiers, also provided a high proportion of university doctors (6.6 per cent) with a further 9.8 per cent in other public sector employment, largely concerned with research. Public sector employment as a whole was highest among St George's Hospital and Westminster Hospital qualifiers (92.5 and 89.2 per cent). Interestingly Nottingham and Southampton, the two new medical schools, contributed least (76.2 per cent), with the exception of Queen's University, Belfast, from which there was a relatively large UK-unknown category.

Grouping of medical schools showed higher NHS employment among graduates of the English provincial schools which were producing doctors in 1974, than from the London teaching hospitals or the Scottish medical schools. However, for the entire public sector, the London medical school group (84.4 per cent) had the largest proportion, and Scottish medical schools the least (80.8 per cent).

For the medical schools which were producing graduates in both 1974 and 1977, the product moment correlation coefficient, *r* (Blalock 1982), for the percentages of qualifiers in NHS employment gave a value of +0.48. This suggests some consistency in the proportions of graduates entering the NHS from different medical schools at equivalent periods of five years after qualifying. It would be interesting to see whether the relationship continued to exist later in doctors' careers, or for those graduating further apart than five years.

There were some clear differences in the numbers of doctors not working, although the overall numbers were small. The largest proportion (7.9 per cent) was from Southampton (five people); this was followed by Bristol (7.1 per cent). Unemployment was marginally greater for the old-established English provincial medical schools and the Scottish medical schools (3.7 per cent) than for the London medical schools (3.0 per cent). Interestingly the group of new provincial medical schools — Cambridge, Nottingham and Southampton — had a reasonably high unemployment rate of 6.4 per cent among their 109 qualifiers. Emigration closely followed the pattern of 1974 qualifiers in 1979. It was highest from the Scottish medical schools, where Edinburgh had 15 per cent of its qualifiers abroad, and Aberdeen 13.9 per cent. The lowest proportions abroad were from St George's Hospital (1.9 per cent of fifty-three qualifiers) and St Mary's Hospital (3.3 per cent). The overall rate for the Scottish medical schools was 11.4 per cent, followed by the old English provincial medical schools with 8.9 per cent and the London medical schools with 7.3 per cent.

As with the previous cohort, a greater percentage of doctors were working in hospital than general practice from all the London medical schools, all the Scottish medical schools (except Glasgow in 1979), and from Birmingham and Bristol. The same was true in 1982 for the newly surveyed schools of Queen's University, Belfast, and Southampton. In contrast, Leeds, Manchester, Newcastle and Sheffield had produced smaller proportions of doctors working in hospital medicine than in general practice on both occasions — thus highlighting the relative popularity of general practice among qualifiers in the north of England, and in 1982 they were joined in this by Oxford and the Nottingham medical school. Interestingly, for individual medical schools, excluding Cambridge because of its small number of qualifiers, the correlation (*r*) between percentages working in general practice five years after qualifying, and the percentages of respondents who gave general practice as a first choice of career in the pre-registration year was +0.69. The strength of the association is in part probably a reflection of the very high persistence of career choices for general practice during the years after qualifying (Chapter 3).

Unemployment

As for the 1974 qualifiers in 1979, higher proportions of women than men were unemployed in all occupation groups. Nevertheless, this later survey showed a large decrease in female unemployment (from 14.2 to 8.9 per cent). This raised the percentage of women employed in all the occupation groups, except in the small non-public sector, which showed a slight fall. For men, the increases seen in the percentages employed in the UK were not explained by a drop in UK unemployment, but by a fall of 3.7 percentage points in the proportion abroad. In contrast, there was actually a small rise in the proportion of women abroad.

Unemployment among women doctors, although proportionately less than for 1974 qualifiers in 1979, was still substantial — in fact the absolute numbers showed little change. At this five-year point in their careers, approximately one in eleven women were not working. The reasons were not surprising, with over three-quarters (seventy-two doctors) mentioning or implying a domestic reason. Other reasons were fairly equal in numbers and included waiting for the next post to start, studying, voluntary unemployment, and illness. Of the twenty unemployed men, fourteen were 'between jobs', five were studying (one for a non-medical career), and one was unable to find work.

The women who were not working had been unemployed for widely varying periods of time up to November 1982, and included one qualifier who had not worked since the pre-registration year. Because of our later surveys, we were able to follow the fortunes of these doctors until 1986. By April of that year, sixty-eight of the ninety-one women doctors who were unemployed in 1982 (74.7 per cent) were known to be medically employed in some capacity either in the UK or abroad. Of the others, one was in non-medical work and six were probably unemployed. Of the twenty men, nineteen had returned to medicine well before April 1986, and the remaining person intended to leave medicine.

DISCUSSION

In terms of high response rates and hence near-completeness, these studies represent a considerable improvement on other studies of doctors' careers and employment status. The usefulness of information of this kind is obvious.

Other studies

Although a number of studies have been made on the employment of women doctors, few have been specifically aimed at estimating their contribution to NHS or public sector medicine, and many studies have concentrated on doctors ten or more years after qualifying. There have, however, been some surveys of doctors approximately five years after qualifying, although the research methods — for example ways of obtaining names and addresses — have differed from ours (Ward *et al.* 1981; Lawrie *et al.* 1966; Flynn and Gardner 1969; Last and Broadie 1970; Scottish Council for Postgraduate Medical Education 1978; Beaumont 1978; Allen 1988).

Ward *et al.* (1981) calculated a 'participation index' for doctors which was analogous to our percentage whole-time equivalent. In most studies the percentage of qualifiers traced was only around 75 per cent and whole-time equivalent calculations have to be made relative to the number of qualifiers traced. An estimate can be made by allocating part-time working half the value of a full-time post; applying the method to Ward's participation index, and to our data, shows such estimates to be reasonable.

In the surveys which concerned only women doctors, there seemed to be a slowly increasing trend in the percentage practising medicine approximately five years after qualifying. Their estimated whole-time equivalent contribution dropped in the early 1960s, but continued to rise through the 1970s, mainly due to an increased proportion of women working full-time. The percentages of men practising, and their whole-time equivalent contributions, from the survey of Last and Broadie (1970), were similar to our own. Higher values were obtained by the Scottish Council for Postgraduate Education (1978): in its survey only 1 man out of 268 was known to be unemployed.

In the surveys of women doctors by Flynn and Gardner (1969) and Beaumont (1978) the percentages of women still practising two to six years after qualifying were rather high, particularly for those in full-time employment. Consequently whole-time equivalent contributions were also high. This may have been because of the more recent graduates included in the samples, but it is also possible that the surveys were not representative of all women doctors, since one concerned graduates of the Royal Free Hospital and the other concerned women doctors in the Thames regions. However, although our data are not sufficiently complete to allow an exact breakdown by medical school, the whole-time equivalent contribution to medicine for 1974 women qualifiers from the Royal Free Hospital in our study was in the range of 55-60 per cent, which is considerably below our overall figure for women in this cohort (67.9 per cent) and the estimate from Flynn and Gardner's data (73 per cent).

Activity and participation

The figures reported for unemployment in the two surveys of this chapter include all doctors who were not working, in either medical or other occupations, at the relevant time. These figures do not, therefore, take into account the fact that many doctors, particularly women, are unavailable for work at certain times, because of other commitments.

The *active stock* of doctors consists of those doctors who are actively seeking employment as well as those employed, although such numbers are often difficult to estimate precisely (Hall 1978). The *inactive stock* comprises 'those doctors who (because of domestic commitments or other reasons) have temporarily dropped out of the active pursuit of medicine, even though they may resume their career later on' (DHSS 1985). There is also the concept of the 'relevant stock' of doctors, which includes those who could potentially return to work in medicine, that is inactive, but not retired doctors. The DHSS Advisory Committee on Medical Manpower Planning (DHSS 1985) used the criterion of doctors who had not been employed in the NHS for five years or more, as a basis for excluding them from the 'relevant stock'.

Our studies offered possible ways of defining which doctors should be included in the active stock, or relevant sock. One method was to study the comments made by respondents about their present situation and future plans. A more formal method, which gave largely similar results, was to identify those known to return to medicine within a maximum of three months after the analysis date on which they were unemployed. We could obtain this information because of the longitudinal nature of our data, and on this criterion fifteen out of twenty men (75.0 per cent) and nineteen among ninety-one women (20.9 per cent) could be deemed part of the 'active stock' — i.e. seeking employment — or part of the 'relevant stock' — i.e. potentially returning to work in medicine.

Activity rates concern the numbers, or percentages, of doctors who are working or potentially working. *Participation rates* take account of part-time working and hence give an indication of the volume of service provided by a given population of doctors.

The 'crude participation rate', already described in relation to whole-time equivalents, takes account of all doctors in the relevant sector. A refinement used in DHSS estimates, is the 'participation rate', which is the average whole-time equivalent per active doctor, that is based on the number of doctors in the 'active stock'.

DHSS estimates

Our figures for 1974 qualifiers in 1979 can be compared with projected stocks of all British-born doctors active in medicine in Great Britain, as estimated in the DHSS Green Paper *Medical Manpower — The Next Twenty Years* (DHSS 1978). At least 95 per cent of our 1974 qualifiers were known to be British-born. Our 1979 whole-time equivalent contribution for men (98.0 per cent) was slightly higher than the DHSS projected percentages for 1975 (97.2) and 1985 (97.3). Our estimated contribution for women was low (68.7 per cent, compared to DHSS figures of 77.1 and 78.8 per cent for 1975 and 1985 respectively). This no doubt reflected the fact that while DHSS figures concern doctors in all age groups, our study concerned women doctors at a time when domestic commitments such as pregnancy and the care of young children are at a high level.

The DHSS Medical Manpower Steering Group (DHSS 1980) reported the whole-time equivalent of British-born and Irish-born civilian doctors working in the NHS during 1974-76 to be about 80 per cent of the total number of active British-born and Irish-born doctors in Great Britain. The Group regarded a range of 80-85 per cent as being a realistic assumption for future projections. From our data, the corresponding percentage for 1974 qualifiers in 1979 was 83.6 per cent — comfortably within the Group's expectations. However, the whole-time equivalent contribution to the NHS in 1979 as a percentage of *all* known 1974 qualifiers was only 69.9 per cent. In other words, the overall wastage due to part-time working, unemployment, non-NHS employment (including university appointments), working in the Armed Forces, and emigration was of the order of 30 per cent. For our 1977 qualifiers in 1982 we included doctors in the Armed Forces as part of the active medical work-force. On this basis, the figure for whole-time NHS contribution was 84.9 per cent. The ratio of NHS work to the population of doctors in the UK had thus increased only marginally. However, the whole-time equivalent contribution of doctors working in the NHS as a percentage of *all* qualifiers increased between our two cohorts from 69.9 to 73.7 per cent, largely because of the smaller proportion of men working abroad, and the movement by women in the UK away from unemployment towards full-time work. Despite considerable change in the UK situation it remained true that at this stage of their careers, approximately the equivalent of two of every ten doctors who were active in the UK were lost from the NHS because they were working part-time, or were not in the NHS. Taking account of those doctors who were unemployed, working abroad, or of unknown occupation, the NHS was employing in 1982 approximately 77 of every 100 doctors who had graduated from UK medical schools five years previously.

Our data can also be compared with the estimates of ACMMP (Advisory Committee on Medical Manpower Planning: DHSS 1985). The 'activity rates' — the ratio of the number of doctors in the active stock to the total 'relevant stock' — were similar for men in our two studies to the ACMMP estimates, but the activity rates of our women doctors were lower, which probably, once again, reflected the fact that our cohorts were still within the child-bearing and child-rearing years. The 'participation rate' for men and women combined was 9.35 for our 1974 qualifiers in 1979, and 9.50 for our 1977 qualifiers in 1982. These figures compared with the ACMMP estimates of 9.42 for 1980 and 9.44 for 1990. The ACMMP estimates offered a range of assumptions, however, and our figure of 9.50 for 1977 qualifiers in 1982 was, in fact, mid-way between their 9.42 estimate and their alternative 1980 'high variant' figure of 9.58.

9 Women doctors

Following a conference at Sunningdale in July 1975, entitled 'Women in Medicine', the DHSS published a draft circular which asked for

> encouragement of all doctors to complete pre-registration training, use of the Doctor Retainer Scheme, re-entry courses, training on a part-time basis, establishment of part-time career posts, planning of needs and opportunities in general practice, and continued career counselling and guidance.
>
> (DHSS 1976)

These sentiments have been repeated so often as to seem mere platitudes, and although there have been numerous, often numerically small, one-off studies there has not been a great deal of continuous longitudinal research. We noted twelve years ago that

> there has never been any systematic monitoring of numbers, choice of career or of career patterns, emigration, and ways of coping with what Celia Oakley (1976) calls 'the same pressures as men plus some obvious additional ones'.
>
> (Parkhouse 1978)

Suggestions for compiling accurate and up-to-date information on a regular, national basis (Parkhouse 1980), for example through an independent institute of medical personnel planning, have not been taken up; political 'necessity' might in any case override inconvenient fact. But we have in our study of a decade of British medical graduates learned a great deal about the women doctors who qualified between 1974 and 1983. The attitudes and work patterns of these women are of great concern to the profession, since in 1960 25 per cent of medical students were women, in 1975 35 per cent, in 1985 46 per cent, and 50 per cent is anticipated for the 1990s.

BACKGROUND INFORMATION

In our studies the proportion of women respondents, at the pre-registration stage, rose from 26.9 per cent of 1974 qualifiers to 39.4 per cent of 1983 qualifiers. In each of our four main cohorts — 1974, 1977, 1980 and 1983 — the response rates were fractionally higher for women than for men.

Many of our findings are reported in other chapters, and they bear out what is well-known and already documented elsewhere — for instance patterns of career choices and sex differences in the rates of part-time work and unemployment. More detail of our women respondents is reported separately (Rhodes 1989a; 1989b; 1989c; 1990).

Tables 9.1 and 9.2 show percentages of women and men who were married, and who had children, in our main cohorts. These figures, like those in other tables, cannot of course reflect the status of non-respondents. It is a persistent problem in studies of women doctors (e.g. Allen 1988) that although very detailed information can be obtained in most cases, the more interesting people to know about are those who have changed their names, given up practice, or decided not to participate. Nevertheless, our response rates were high, and it is obvious that at all stages after qualifying, higher proportions of men than women were married, and higher proportions had children. It is also very obvious that the timing of marriage and starting a family was later, for both men and women, among the more recent qualifiers.

Career choices of men and women respondents are given in Chapter 3. The fact that fewer women respondents than men made firm career choices at the pre-registration stage may be due to existing domestic commitments which bear more heavily on women than men, on uncertainty about future domestic commitments which may frustrate ambitions, or the belief that it is harder for women than men to succeed in some specialties, for various reasons (Rhodes 1989a; Allen 1988). Some women may prefer less popular specialties, and some may find competitiveness unappealing (Wills 1986). Among our 1974 and 1977 respondents, women with children were least likely to give definite choices at three, five and seven years after qualifying, while men with children were the most likely to do so. Married respondents in these two cohorts were more likely to choose general practice than single doctors, and those with children more likely to do so than those with none; in each case the tendency was most marked among women. Community medicine and community health, although given as choices by relatively

Table 9.1 Percentage of women married at time of reply compared with men

		Years after qualifying						
Year of qualifying		*1 year*	*3 years*	*5 years*	*7 years*	*9 years*	*11 years*	*13 years*
1974	Women	41.1	60.8	67.8	72.6	79.0	76.7	78.7
	Men	42.4	70.1	76.6	82.9	86.0	87.4	90.7
1977	Women	32.8	51.9	64.5	72.3	74.9		
	Men	34.7	57.8	70.9	80.5	85.2		
1980	Women	21.1	43.7	58.6				
	Men	23.5	48.3	65.5				
1983	Women	20.5	38.9					
	Men	20.8	44.2					

Table 9.2 Percentage of women with children at time of reply compared with men[a]

Year of qualifying		*Years after qualifying*						
		1 year	*3 years*	*5 years*	*7 years*	*9 years*	*11 years*	*13 years*
1974	Women		18.6	40.1	55.3	66.1	70.8	77.6
	Men		29.7	51.5	64.6	72.6	81.4	86.1
1977	Women		9.4	27.0	48.6	55.7		
	Men		16.7	39.1	56.4	71.3		
1980	Women	1.7	6.1	21.1				
	Men	4.4	12.5	32.3				
1983	Women	1.9	7.4					
	Men	3.8	11.9					

Note: a The 1974 cohort was not asked this question in 1975, nor the 1977 cohort in 1978

Table 9.3 Percentages of respondents, by sex, holding posts in some major specialties and grades

	General practice									
	Total	*Prin.*	*Asst*	*Surg.*	*Med.*	*Comm. Med.*	*Reg.*	*SR*	*Cons.*	*Academic*
1974 cohort in 1987										
Men	32.4	24.6	0.6	11.0	10.3	1.3	1.0	6.2	20.3	5.6
Women	32.7	22.2	5.6	2.3	5.2	6.0	0.7	4.7	11.4	3.3
1977 cohort in 1986										
Men	33.5	28.7	1.1	11.6	10.1	1.1	5.6	14.6	7.5	8.1
Women	32.0	21.3	7.2	2.6	5.6	5.7	4.3	9.3	5.3	4.2
1980 cohort in 1985										
Men	26.6	17.0	7.8	12.0	11.6	0.9	24.3	3.6	0.1	5.5
Women	28.5	13.8	12.5	3.5	4.3	5.6	18.9	3.7	0.1	2.9
1983 cohort in 1986										
Men	9.8	0.1	8.1	16.7	20.7	0.4	11.1	0.1		1.9
Women	10.9	0.1	10.1	9.7	16.2	1.5	7.3	0.1		1.0

few respondents, were about equally popular among men and women who were single, but much more popular among married women, especially those with children, and much less popular among married men. Medicine and surgery were least popular among respondents with children and, for women, marriage was clearly associated with a decision against choosing surgery or, to a lesser extent, medicine. Seven years after qualifying, the popularity of medicine and surgery remained fairly similar for single and married men (Rhodes 1989a).

Table 9.3 shows the types and grades of post held by women respondents from our main cohorts, compared with men, at the times of their latest replies to us. The picture shows the disparity in numbers between men and women working in medicine and surgery, and the greater numbers of women in community medicine. Proportionately fewer women than men had become consultants, and fewer had obtained academic posts. In general practice, women were more likely than men to be assistants rather than principals. It has been suggested that the changes recently proposed by the Secretary of State for Health, Mr Kenneth Clarke, would make it advantageous for practices to employ women doctors part-time as assistants rather than making them partners; they would then be used for work such as cervical cancer screening and childhood immunization, to secure the income attracted by the new arrangements, without having any direct influence on the way the practice operates (Harman 1989). The BMA Conference of 1989 declared that action must be taken to break down the barriers that keep women out of top jobs in the NHS, discrimination existing to the extent that all of the forty-four consultant general surgeons appointed in the period 1984-9 were men. The conference endorsed their Working Party's recommendations for more part-time training opportunities, child-care provision, a campaign for child-care expenses to be tax deductible, and a requirement that health authorities meet targets on employing women doctors (BMA 1989). Which all seems to be where we came in!

PART-TIME WORK AND UNEMPLOYMENT

The general employment picture emerging from our studies is partly described in Chapter 8, and some specific aspects are dealt with in Chapters 10-14 on individual specialties.

Some problems arise in defining part-time work and unemployment. In general practice, 'sessions' are not described and exact hours worked may not be stated (Chapter 14). It is sometimes hard to know if a doctor is actually working part-time, especially as other commitments that go with general practice (such as police, school or factory work) may not be mentioned. Very often our respondents had two or more part-time jobs concurrently, and the overlapping of various commitments might be complex, so that within a year or so of mixed commitments there might be a few weeks here and there of genuinely part-time work. In fact, however, detailed analysis of a sample of our respondents (Rhodes 1990) showed that for each of the women in the sample the sum total of work during the 'part-time' period was actually less than full-time, whereas the only man in the sample had used the balance of his time in other employment. Unless a specific sessional commitment is declared, and it is clear that no other medical work was involved, there will always be a margin of doubt in any assessment of the true extent of part-time work — a more detailed view of this for our 1974 and 1977 respondents is given by Rhodes (1990).

There are various definitions of unemployment (see Chapter 8). The official government definition based on numbers receiving benefit is open to various criticisms, and is in any case largely inapplicable to the situation in medicine. Self-reporting of unemployment among our respondents ranged from those who left long unexplained gaps between their listed jobs, to those who pointed out gaps of three or four days by underlining the word unemployment twice. Periods of apparent unemployment in a questionnaire reply often disappeared in subsequent replies by elision of dates. Some breaks between jobs were obviously regarded as natural, or inevitable, and quite frequently welcome. Indeed, the voluntary nature of a period without work was sometimes clearly stated.

For both part-time working and unemployment the levels reported will depend on the minimum time considered reasonable — e.g. periods of three months or more working part-time or unemployed (Rhodes 1989b; 1990). More searching criteria can be applied by including shorter periods; different groups of doctors can be compared only if the same criteria are used.

We looked at women who qualified in 1974, taking those who replied to us in 1987 and adding in usable information from the earlier replies of some who did not respond in 1987. Our purpose was to relate part-time work and employment to family size. Thus, in this analysis, although jobs held and reported periods of part-time work or unemployment do not relate to a specific date, they always relate to the number of children that respondents had at the time. All gaps between jobs, however short, are included as unemployment, and all part-time posts, however

Table 9.4 Respondents by number of children and latest known employment (1974 qualifiers)

			Latest known medical work						
No. of children	*No. (%) of respondents*		*Full-time*	*(%)*	*Part-time*	*(%)*	*None*	*(%)*	*Unknown*
None	144	(24)	120	(83)	19	(13)	2	(1)	3
1	78	(13)	33	(42)	38	(49)	4	(5)	3
2	224	(37)	73	(33)	124	(55)	24	(11)	3
3	119	(20)	17[a]	(14)	80	(67)	15[b]	(13)	7
3+	36	(6)	4	(11)	23	(64)	6	(17)	3
Total	601	(100)	247	(41)	284	(47)	51	(8)	19

Notes: a Including one dentist
b Including one deceased

brief, are included. If there was residual doubt about whether the total commitment from two or more jobs was full-time or part-time, the case was entered in the last column of Table 9.4.

Table 9.4 shows that this analysis includes 601 women doctors, of whom 24 per cent had no children. Having two children was the commonest state of affairs (37 per cent); 26 per cent had three or more children at the time of their latest replies. Although 83 per cent of those with no children were working full-time, this proportion was almost halved, to 42 per cent, among those with only one child. Only 14 per cent of those with three or more children were working full-time, but only 14 per cent were not working at all. Nearly half of all the women surveyed (47 per cent), and half to two-thirds of all those with children, were doing part-time jobs.

Tables 9.5 and 9.6 give details of unemployment and part-time work, from graduation up to and including the time of the latest reply and the current job at that point, for women doctors from medical schools in Scotland, the English provinces and Wales, and London, according to the number of children. In these tables part-time jobs prior to the latest known job are included whether or not they were held concurrently with other jobs.

Table 9.5 Percentages of respondents with periods of unemployment and part-time work, with cumulated total numbers of periods of unemployment and part-time work per 100 respondents (1974 qualifiers)[a]

		Unemployment			
No. of children	*Medical school group*	*1 or 2 periods*	*3 or more periods*	*total % of respondents*	*total periods per 100 respondents*
None	Scotland	25	0	25	32
	English provincial and Wales	35	4	39	60
	London	41	11	52	107
	Total	35	5	40	69
1 or 2	Scotland	42	22	64	136
	English provincial and Wales	37	20	57	121
	London	46	23	69	149
	Total	42	22	63	136
3 or more	Scotland	52	24	76	179
	English provincial and Wales	51	28	79	162
	London	51	25	75	159
	Total	51	26	77	165

Note: a See Table 9.6

The figures in Table 9.5 are percentages of respondents who had had various numbers of periods of unemployment and part-time work, and the cumulative total number of periods of each, per hundred doctors, is shown in order to relate to Table 9.6. The two halves of the table are not mutually exclusive, since many respondents had worked part-time and also been unemployed.

Even with no children, 40 per cent of women had been unemployed at some stage and 25 per cent had held at least one part-time job. Both unemployment and part-time work were strongly influenced by family size (chi-square comparisons between pairs of totals, $p < 0.05$ to < 0.001). The incidence of unemployment among London women qualifiers with no children was significantly higher than among Scottish women qualifiers with no children ($p < 0.05$).

Part-time work			
1 or 2 periods	*3 or more periods*	*total % of respondents*	*total periods per 100 respondents*
7	7	15	43
24	4	28	49
16	11	27	57
18	7	25	50
29	48	77	258
39	34	73	192
42	38	80	209
37	39	76	216
39	55	94	321
33	56	89	308
31	49	80	279
34	53	86	299

Table 9.6 gives an analysis of individual periods of unemployment and part-time work, by duration, expressed as the rate per hundred doctors. For women doctors with no children there was, on average, one part-time job for every two doctors, for those with one or two children there were just over two part-time jobs per doctor and for those with three or more children there were three part-time jobs per doctor. This relationship to family size also applied to unemployment. The commonest durations of unemployment and part-time work shifted notably towards periods of more than six months among those with children; in fact, for women with more than three children there were fifty-three periods of unemployment of more than a year and 144 periods of part-time work of more than a year per hundred doctors.

Table 9.6 Rates of unemployment and part-time work per 100 respondents, by duration (1974 qualifiers)

		Unemployment			*Part-time work*		
No. of children	*Medical school group*	*less than 6 months*	*6 months or more*	*total incl. ?*	*less than 6 months*	*6 months or more*	*total incl. ?*
None	Scotland	21	7	32	0	29	43
	English provincial and Wales	53	3	60	13	19	49
	London	84	20	107	18	23	57
	Total	56	9	69	12	22	50
1 or 2	Scotland	56	55	136	36	151	258
	English provincial and Wales	47	58	121	28	101	192
	London	75 •	47	149	24	113	209
	Total	60	53	136	28	118	216
3 or more	Scotland	52	79	179	30	194	321
	English provincial and Wales	64	64	162	38	170	308
	London	54	69	159	51	131	279
	Total	57	69	165	41	160	299

Tables 9.5 and 9.6 together show that unemployment among women doctors with no children tended to be short-term and non-recurrent and this is confirmed by inspection of individual replies from respondents. Also, the much higher incidence of unemployment among London women qualifiers with no children than among others with no children, particularly from Scottish medical schools, is again seen in Table 9.6.

Family size varies with fashion, among many other factors, and medical work patterns depend on a complex interplay of supply and demand for full- and part-time jobs. The information given here complements other, more general reports on women doctors' career plans and employment from our studies (Rhodes 1989a; 1989b; 1990) and elsewhere, and analyses of the employment position of British doctors of both sexes (Parkhouse *et al.* 1982; Ellin and Parkhouse 1989). The picture is one of coping with the dual responsibilities of bringing up children and continuing with medical practice. It clearly shows not only the extent to which women doctors seek and depend on part-time work as family size increases, but also the extent to which many facets of the work of the NHS depend on the availability of part-time doctors. These are complementary facts that we ignore at our peril, with a changing ethos of working life and family commitment, among both men and women, and an increasing proportion of women in medicine.

Reasons given for unemployment may not accurately reflect the private thoughts of the respondent. Domestic circumstances may be considered a more socially acceptable reason by women than by men, although those women who are worried by the economic arguments against enrolling female medical students may wish to play these reasons down. Some respondents doubtless thought about the uses that might be made of our data, and some certainly took advantage of the chance to express their frustrations. The reasons that seem most important in retrospect might not have been the most powerful motivating forces at the time. Reasons are often complex; a move may come for various purposes, and may then lead to long-term unemployment for other reasons; a forced career break may lead to declining ambition or be seen as a good time to start a family.

Among 1974 and 1977 respondents, there were 189 women and 28 men who reported periods of one year or more during which they were not working in medicine. Among the women, domestic commitments including pregnancy and child-care were given as reasons by 121 (64.0 per cent). The next commonest reason was move with a husband (21.2 per cent) and in more than half of the cases (11.6 per cent) this was associated with

Table 9.7 The 1974 qualifiers in 1987

Medical school	*Questionnaires sent* *total*	*to women*	*No. of women who replied*
Aberdeen	97	37	32
Birmingham	119	34	30
Bristol	89	32	31
Dundee	65	20	16
Edinburgh	143	34	28
Glasgow	187	56	38
Leeds	72	21	16
Liverpool	118	32	27
Manchester	145	46	36
Newcastle	77	23	20
Oxford	45	7	5
Sheffield	79	25	19
Wales	90	26	24
Charing Cross	40	10	8
Guy's	115	17	12
King's College	81	20	17
The London	112	20	14
Middlesex	82	13	13
Royal Free	89	42	35
St Bart's	83	12	10
St George's	61	11	9
St Mary's	82	25	21
St Thomas'	78	14	13
UCH	105	31	27
Westminster	69	13	9
Total	2,323	621 (26.7%)	510 (82.13%)

Source: Parkhouse and Parkhouse 1989a

pregnancy. 'No suitable job' was the next commonest reason, given by 12.7 per cent of these women respondents. Among the relatively few men, the commonest reasons given for unemployment were travel, ill-health or study (53.6 per cent altogether) and only one man gave domestic reasons. The commonest combination of reasons among women respondents (11.6 per cent) was pregnancy and/or care of children with lack of a suitable job (Rhodes 1989c).

THE 1974 QUALIFIERS: WOMEN'S VIEWS

The questionnaire we sent to 1974 qualifiers in 1987 included a special supplement for women doctors asking for a voluntary evaluation of career progress, an assessment of future trends, and advice to women doctors now qualifying. Of 2,323 questionnaires sent, 621 went to women doctors and replies were received from 510 (82.1 per cent). The breakdown by medical school is given in Table 9.7. Their comments illustrate very well the range of issues which have been discussed over the years.

Comments concern both the family and work. Family comments were in three main areas. First, husband's job: a non-medical or GP spouse presented fewer problems than a specialist in training, and the need for a supportive attitude, in practice as well as theoretically, was important. The geographical factor of having to move with husband's work (or being unable to move because of it) caused many problems. Second, children: when or if to have them, whether to take time off only for maternity leave, or until the children start school, or longer. Third, the need for domestic cover and its varying availability, the need for tax relief, and feelings of guilt because of using a substitute at home. With regard to work, comments concerned the inadequacy of careers counselling and the need for it from school to the postgraduate level; the necessity of achieving postgraduate examinations before starting a family; the importance of part-time training and later part-time work; the difficulties and advantages of job sharing; and pros and cons of the Retainer Scheme; the advantages of general practice in terms of flexibility, and patient contact; the difficulties with over-subscribed specialties compared to careers in geriatrics and psychiatry, community health, etc.; attitudes, now changing, towards married women with children (single women found no discrimination); and the need for job satisfaction in whatever work is chosen.

Table 9.8 shows the relative importance attached to various factors by the 510 women who responded with comments. Almost 40 per cent of these respondents commented on the importance of their husband's work; over a third were concerned about responsibilities to their family; 27 per cent remarked on the suitability of general practice as a career and 15 per cent stressed the importance of obtaining postgraduate qualifications before starting a family. Without prompting, 20 per cent said that they were currently happy with their work; only 2.6 per cent said that, given their time over again, they would not become doctors.

Table 9.8 Relative importance of various factors to women respondents (1974 qualifiers)

Factors influencing career paths			*% of respondents commenting*	
Domestic				
Husband				
– spouse's work			38.4	
– supportive attitude of spouse			9.8	
– geographical	– tied		5.1	
	– moving		15.7	
Single/no children			3.3	
Children				
– responsibility to family			33.9	
– need for domestic help			9.6	
– finance			8.0	
– feelings of guilt			1.2	
Career				
Need for	– careers advice		7.1	
	– careers planning		3.5	
	– clinical updating		1.6	
Retainer Scheme	– for		5.5	7.3
	– against		1.8	
Maternity leave			5.7	
Obtaining qualifications before family			14.9	
Part-time training	– for		11.0	12.6
	– against		1.6	
Part-time work	– for		19.4	20.0
	– against		0.6	
Job sharing			7.8	
GP suitable for women			26.9	
Other specialties suitable for women			15.5	
Difficulties of hospital career			4.9	
Attitude of male colleagues		– negative	7.7	15.9
		– neutral	4.3	
		– positive	3.9	
Job satisfaction			20.4	
Would not do medicine again			2.6	

Source: Parkhouse and Parkhouse 1989a

Altogether, if broken down under the headings of Table 9.8, there were 1,487 comments from these doctors. Of these comments, 42 per cent related to husbands and children and, most commonly among career factors, 9 per cent referred to general practice. There were seventy-nine comments about the suitability for women of careers other than general practice. Nineteen of these related to community health, community paediatrics, community psychiatry and family planning, eleven were for various branches of psychiatry and ten for pathology specialties. Mentioned five or six times were dermatology, geriatrics and anaesthetics.

This précis can be set alongside recent publications, and illustrated with some individual respondents' comments — as trenchant and well expressed as one would expect from the scholastic high-flyers who enter medicine.

Equality and equal opportunity

Lefford (1987) said 'Equal opportunity for entry to medicine is in sight. Can the same be said of the career opportunities for women doctors?' In 1969 9 per cent of medical students were women. In 1987 37 per cent of the first-year medical students were women and, of course, the percentage is still rising. But although the proportion of women in junior NHS grades has closely followed the rise in proportion of graduates, the number of consultants, typically, has not, even allowing for the time lag. 'The higher the level one looks in a profession, the smaller proportion of women will be found' (Epstein and Coeser 1982); and 'women are not proportionately distributed throughout all specialties' (Berliner 1988). Their numbers in surgery and medicine have not really changed, and a meeting in London of women gynaecologists in 1987 (Gillie 1988) reported that the number of women becoming consultants had not increased in the last twenty-five years although the number of women doctors had increased four-fold. 'The profession needs restructuring: one in five men and women specialising in obstetrics and gynaecology later regretted it because the job is so demanding.' So perhaps men, as well as women, require change in the career structure and work patterns.

Lefford goes on:

> There is no evidence of different intellectual or psychomotor skills — the female entrants to medical school are potential high fliers, so why the under-achievement? The preference

> for domestic commitment may be true for some women some of the time; it is not true for most women doctors most of their lifetime. The present career structure of postgraduate training coincides with women's optimum reproductive period so part-time training is essential and flexibility in work patterns is needed.
>
> (Lefford 1987)

Lorber commented that

> numbers alone are not the answer to gender inequality — it depends where the power goes. There is a need for professional networking and support groups, and senior women must help the career advancement of younger women. The ultimate goal is not to join the inner circles imbued with the male perspective on work, family life and social service, but for the establishment of new values which reflect the needs and priorities of all members of society.
>
> (Lorber 1984)

One of our respondents wrote:

> appointment committees seem to like appointing people like themselves, i.e. white, male, middle-class. There are far more women consultants in the non-teaching districts, and therefore few role models for female students in the teaching districts.

Discrimination

Discrimination against women doctors, and the consequent need for patronage, was not an important factor for the women respondents in this 1974 cohort, although one said,

> at the end of house jobs the consultant for whom I worked refused to give all women housemen a reference for general medicine or general surgery: that type of bigotry is going slowly.

But there is still a feeling that women need to prove themselves.

> I have come across very little overt chauvinism towards me as a woman by my male colleagues but I feel I must work hard at ensuring that I do a good job, equal and sometimes

> better in competence, than them,

which is a pity.

Specialty differences

General practice, as with men, is a favourite choice because it allows time for home and family:

> I find the flexible timing of work schedule suits my domestic arrangements. I also feel a definite role in the partnership because of being a woman, in the realm of obstetrics and gynaecology in particular.

Others consider that there is still exploitation of women in general practice:

> Plenty of GPs regard women doctors as cheap labour and think we should be glad of it — don't put up with it! After six years I said to the partners — 'I do an equal share of work and receive a third of your incomes as salaried partners — some improvement would only be fair' — they said it had been nice working with me.

She was geographically tied because of her husband's career but found another practice:

> Less hours, opinions on organization, finance, etc. considered equally with other partners, special interests developed (e.g. diabetic clinic) and income geared to rise to pro rata parity.

Perhaps this is not all one-sided:

> I enjoy the flexible hours and the opportunity to opt out of out-of-hours work because this suits my domestic and other commitments. I have had problems with partnerships because of this.

And one with more of a conscience:

> I seem to be absent from decision-making meetings because of family commitments — I hope this will be less problematic as the children get older.

And a plea for longer maternity leave:

> only thirteen weeks in total which means working until thirty-seven or thirty-eight weeks prior to the birth to get reasonable time off afterwards.

Psychiatry was regarded as 'a good specialty for women with families because few night calls and flexible hours'. A staff anaesthetist respondent, at present in Canada, reported:

> I can job share with little detriment to patients and colleagues, and have a career that will travel with husband's requirements.

Others have left hospital work:

> I loved being charged up in hectic acute work but found it difficult to balance the rest of my life.

A consultant in obstetrics and gynaecology, who was single, wrote:

> It would be virtually impossible to progress as I did and expect to have any children until achieving consultant status or at least senior registrar level.

Another respondent

> wanted to be a gynaecologist but compromised with radiology because wanted large family — now specialist in diagnostic ultrasound with hours 8 a.m. to 3 p.m. (in Israel)

Careers counselling

The need for careers counselling was widely felt, and from the outset, prior to embarking on a medical career:

> As someone who had no medical background I had little idea of what was ahead of me other than six years at university, and received no guidance.

> I could have used my time more efficiently had I made an earlier career decision and not tried various options.

And in moving with their husbands round the country, women need career advice in the new region — only one in the cohort praised a Postgraduate Dean for helping her to find a new career in London after five years as a rural GP.

Part-time training and the Retainer Scheme

Ward (1982) found that over 90 per cent of women graduates from UK medical schools in 1949, 1951 and 1965 were practising in 1977 — a higher rate of professional activity than any other professional group (dentists 85 per cent, nurses 51 per cent, teachers 41 per cent), but she questioned the quality of work and concluded that more women than men fail to reach their full potential as medical practitioners. Part-time training and work, and job sharing, arouse very different reactions:

> Those people who are usually supernumeraries get to choose what they want to do and don't do all the unwanted work.
>
> There is a lack as regards patient follow-up unless the doctor is motivated to do this.
>
> The slow progress of part-time training is demoralizing.
>
> Lack of part-time posts in NE Scotland, compared with Southern England.
>
> Part-time and job-sharing posts are useful and should be integrated within most medical departments, accepting that in order to perform the job more time will be needed than is contracted.

That seems reasonable, it being the case with all part-time jobs, but what of this comment?

> If women doctors train part-time (and with a couple of notable exceptions the part-time women I have met are not as good or as dedicated as the men) they must prove that they are exceptional if they wish to gain the support of their male colleagues.

The same doctor (no children) goes on:

> Children if they exist must not intrude on work. Adequate

child care is necessary and may result in significant expense.

One doctor wrote:

> I would like to see develop in medicine more part-time work and job sharing, not just for women; perhaps some male doctors would like two part-time jobs rather than work all their days in one narrow field.

(Nicol 1987) quoted a survey of 500 patients in an Edinburgh practice which showed that patients of job-sharing doctors were seen faster and found them more 'available' than full-time partners, and 25 per cent of the Edinburgh patients specifically asked to see a woman doctor. As far back as 1966 Jean Lawrie was writing:

> Health Services should adopt a more flexible attitude to part-time workers and, as well as at the consultant level, opportunities for part-time employment and study should be available in all grades. Social factors which affect the employment of all professional women should be urgently examined.
>
> (Lawrie *et al*. 1966)

Egerton (1987) listed the advantages of women doctors over other working women.

> The Retainer Scheme is singular among the professions: it facilitates women who stop work completely during the child-raising period.

Attitudes to the Retainer Scheme vary:

> Married women whose husbands require to move frequently for career advancement must be very adaptable if their husband's career is priority (which is often the case when children are young). The Doctor Retainer Scheme has helped greatly in introducing me to new practices as we moved around.

> Moving with my husband it was possible to plan training jobs and I completed my vocational training and MRCGP exams before having my family [but she concludes] I think the Doctor Retainer Scheme is a bit of a farce.

One doctor wrote:

> The Doctor Retainer Scheme allowed me to keep skills up to date.

Another said:

> I had to leave to work more than two sessions.

The reality is that most women build up their work as the family grows up — so why not have a scheme that reflects and encourages this?

> I feel slightly trapped, I would like to increase hours (for example Clinical Assistant (CA) sessions) but would have to leave Scheme.

> I wish refresher courses were incorporated into the Retainer Scheme: getting back is hard, prescribing is a major headache when you haven't done it for many years.

> Reading can be done alone but I didn't find a safe area to refresh clinical skills.

Some find unemployment (whether for reasons of children or moving) a problem: 'morale lowering and very boring'; another respondent, however, said:

> I found taking time out a positive advantage in that it gave me a different perspective on the career ladder.

Finance

Finance often seems to pose a problem because of the high standard of domestic and child-care required.

> Be prepared to allocate large proportion of income for reliable child-care, otherwise emotional strain unbearable.

> I need to work full-time because of cost of nanny and housekeeper, plus taxes, plus Medical Defence Union fees rising astronomically would otherwise leave barely any earnings.

Earnings are however high compared to most other working

women:

> General practice (with flexible hours, freedom from hierarchy and chance to develop my own interests) provides a good enough income for my husband to stay at home and look after our baby while I have returned to work.

And as women often marry within the profession,

> I have no financial need to work, I have taken up teaching as it fits in with the children's holidays and is far less stressful. I can pick up medicine again if there is economic need.

Not very many other women can say:

> Early on I decided that career would be secondary to other aspects of my life, I have travelled widely, lived overseas and enjoy looking after our daughter.

A GP respondent, married with one child, wrote:

> I am the family breadwinner: what other job can do that for a woman, part-time?

Social factors

An Australian study concluded

> Women have more role conflict and less role support as their medical training progresses. The development of interpersonal relations with mentors and colleagues is restricted to men so women are excluded from peer activities. Exclusion from informal networks reduces women's ability to operate within the power structure and may virtually eliminate the methods by which some students attain sponsorships into higher status positions. In addition there are the special problems experienced by women who choose to marry. A question that needs to be investigated concerns the extent to which they achieve the goals and aspirations they see for themselves; are they disadvantaged in their attempt to move into specialty and postgraduate programmes?
> (Shapiro *et al.* 1988)

Social factors include the role of husbands, who are commonly referred to as being very supportive:

> I have found no difficulties incorporating motherhood into my career (GP), my husband takes a very positive and helpful attitude.

But,

> A woman still has to do two jobs if she wants a career. Men don't do equal shares of the mundane; problems regarding children, nanny, school runs all fall on me.

> I take on all the commitments to the small rural community and local primary school, e.g. school council, PTA, Guides and Brownies, etc. My husband does not have time for these.

This is echoed by 'Consideration of the husband's career is important' and 'Husband's career must not be jeopardized'. And on moving:

> Having moved round the world with my husband in the Armed Forces, my career is in shambles; there are virtually no training prospects for civilian wives with the army, just filling in wherever a vacancy arises. The money is reasonably good but career prospects virtually nil.

> Moving to West Germany with spouse I found my MRC Psych not accepted and I must complete two-years neurology full-time on call. This was impossible with children and my career prospects are miserable.

Even in the UK the situation is very variable:

> Husband a GP (on a remote island), very little choice of work.

> Husband's work in Northern Scotland, cannot find part-time work therefore am reading law.

Alternatively

> Husband a consultant in central London therefore a consultant job-share is a realistic possibility because of the increased geographical area.

Since many women arrange their careers around the family — 'GP to fit in with the family' and 'Husband believes in his own career priority' — it may be that the supportiveness of the husband's role is not always put fully to the test.

> On the family issue
>
> Family commitments appear to be regarded as a stabilizing influence on men but a lack of career commitment for a woman.
>
> Commitments to children over-ride all other obstacles women have to face in medicine. Good child-care facilities must exist so that women can divide themselves without guilt.

One respondent put it forcibly:

> The news that 'Mum's on duty' meets with groans of 'Not again', and seems to cause more problems than Dad's disappearing for days at a time.

Another regretted

> building up my career around my husband's job location rather than medical centres of excellence.

The feminine contribution to medicine

The NHS is the largest employer of women in Britain today — 75 per cent of its work-force are women, congregated in certain occupations and at particular status levels, nurses, clerical, and ancillary staff (a large number are migrant and ethnic minority workers — again the majority are women) 'an environment deeply divided in gender terms, a situation richly patterned with gender assumptions and institutionalised patriarchal power relations' (Doyal *et al.* 1980). Spencer and Podmore in *In a Man's World* wrote:

> Women are directed towards aspects of professional work where a large measure of traditional feminine qualities are required, that is helping, caring, giving social and emotional support — what has been called women's stroking function.
>
> (Spencer and Podmore 1987)

The *Guardian* published a letter saying

> One of the commonest requests to the FPC is for the name of a practice with a female partner as for some women discussing intimate problems or having intimate examinations is less easy if the doctor is male.
>
> (Singleton 1988)

As attitudes, expectations and opportunities continue to change in society and in medicine — and they will as more women enter the profession — then, as Berliner observed, 'patients will begin to experience a different nature of interaction with their doctors than they have traditionally received' (Berliner 1988). This must have implications for job-sharing and the full participation of women in the team, at all levels. Optimum medical care is the goal; Enoch Powell, in 1966, wrote

> In the hospital service (as compared with the Armed Forces) there is no single aim that can be formulated . . . the whole activity is, and ought to be, the sum of individual and personal judgements, not orientated towards the centre, but outwards to the individual patient.
>
> (Powell 1966)

Job satisfaction

> My children and my husband's job have affected my choice of career (GP) but I have always been conscious that the career choice which I have made needs to be one that will be fulfilling for the rest of my working life.

> Job satisfaction can still be very great even with part-time.

More ambiguously:

> A job is what you make it. Once in a job one should always be able to find areas to enjoy.

And more straightforwardly:

> I'd say go for what you want and hang on to it. That includes opting for part-time work, husband and family, if you want it, and say go hang to the superwoman careerists.

But, for those who want to pursue a specialty and

> progress well and then find keeping up incompatible with having a family, getting back is very difficult and the profession as a whole requires to consider the problem more seriously. Otherwise there will continue to be considerable lost potential for the individuals concerned and for the Health Service.

These comments on job satisfaction come from women doctors at a particular stage of their careers and family lives, and this is a point which requires considerable emphasis. Our surveys have concerned doctors qualifying between 1974 and 1983, and we have followed them for periods of up to thirteen years from leaving medical school. Further questionnaires sent in fifteen or twenty years' time would no doubt bring forth a variety of different comments about medical and social choices, and their consequences, from both men and women.

Comment

The great majority of the women in our 1974 cohort were content, at present, with their work:

> I am very happy with my present job although I do realize that it is a non-training grade, a fact I may regret in the future when the children have grown up, especially if I have to become the main breadwinner in the family for any reason.

Probably this point would not have been considered by an earlier generation, and would have been taken for granted by more recent qualifiers. In fact, the 1974 cohort seems an 'in between' one: a reflection of women in society as a whole, of which they are a part: very nearly all working, but half part-time, satisfied at present with their work yet not achieving their full career potential.

A decade before, family responsibilities would, for most, have meant less work and a feeling of dependence on patronage in an unequal society. Our later (1983) qualifiers, by contrast, seem far more confident about their own abilities, but then nearly 50 per cent of that cohort are women and the time is perceived (although not yet achieved) when half the medical work-force will be women. Guilt feelings about working part-time or in blocks will no doubt pass; other university faculties have long courses, many students stay on for research, and postgraduate training is not uncommon. Yet because many non-medical graduates cannot find work in their own field they change direction and retrain, as all the work-force must be prepared to do nowadays. Medicine, traditionally a discipline apart, is becoming more specialized within itself as technology advances and is not yet flexible enough in combining with other professions; although a great strength of general practice lies in beginning to do just that, in teams with other health and social workers — one reason why it is so attractive to women.

The replies to our questionnaires demonstrated, naturally, a great variety of attitudes, yet a pattern emerged of common factors, of widely felt priorities: the feeling of the need to 'achieve a balance', that it is a woman's responsibility to contain successfully both aspects of her life, domestic and career. There is a responsibility for the family: a wish to support her husband's career, the need to have work that can be coped with as part of life, not to waste medical training, feeling not part of the traditional male medical establishment, and a desire for patient contact.

In inviting the comments from women doctors which gave substance to this survey, we prompted a little, if indirectly, by saying

> Some relevant points may be: attitudes in the medical profession; children; husband's work; part-time/full-time training; job satisfaction; difficulties in some specialties, and some geographical areas. etc.

Despite this potential bias towards unfavourable comment, there were some striking differences between our responses and those reported in Isobel Allen's large study (Allen 1988), particularly in the generally more optimistic tone of our replies, the lower emphasis on 'patronage' and the very few respondents who felt thoroughly disillusioned with medicine as a career.

Evaluating the views, hopes and frustrations of women doctors, in general and in particular, is no easy task; the shades of emphasis in response to face-to-face enquiry from a team of non-medical, all-women interviewers with prestructured questions is likely to be quite different from that elicited by an open-ended written enquiry from a neutral but, we hope, familiar and comfortably regarded research group, and different again from the responses given to a local or national figure with potential influence in appointment committees and reviews concerning promotion. An important factor is that people who at the age of 30, with a pleasant home and two young children, are contented with their professional work may feel differently twenty years later.

What is needed to give career 'fulfilment' to a highly intelligent and very well trained modern British doctor depends on personality at least as much as intellect, and in a multifaceted profession this is just as well when remembering what doctors are for. Comprehensive medical care for the public needs technical wizardry and academic brilliance as well as holistic practice; hard-drivers as well as those who have time to stand and stare; and we have ample evidence from our surveys that the graduates of our medical schools can find fulfilment in all these ways.

Women doctors voice many of the feelings of women in general, and of doctors in general. Comparisons have been made with women in other professions (Fogarty *et al.* 1981), which certainly do not suggest that women doctors are relatively disadvantaged; there is no doubt that men doctors have many of the same grumbles as women about the organization of their profession, and the attitudes within it. The recommendations that are currently made to alleviate the lot of women doctors are merely palliative; cure is a far-reaching concept, for the whole medical profession and society.

10 Individual specialties
Medicine

The term 'medicine' is used in this context to comprise general medicine and all the 'medical' specialties shown in the tables for this chapter (see Table 10.1). It therefore includes, for example, communicable diseases, genito-urinary medicine, haematology, and tropical medicine, but does not include paediatrics or occupational health. The term 'general medicine' is used to include all respondents who gave their career choices or jobs as 'medicine', 'general medicine', 'academic medicine', or medicine/general medicine with a special interest, for example in gastroenterology or diabetes. 'Other medicine' includes doctors who specified career choices or jobs in allergy, aviation medicine, metabolic medicine, nutrition, sports medicine, terminal care, and underwater medicine.

In this and the following chapters on individual specialties, information is based on respondents who qualified in 1974 and 1977 (Parkhouse and Ellin 1990 b-e).

CAREER CHOICES

Table 10.1 shows the percentages of respondents giving various branches of medicine as their first choice of career at different times after qualifying. It shows the striking decline in the number of choices, as the years go by, already noted in Chapter 3, and demonstrates that this falling off is almost entirely due to the reduced number of choices for general medicine. Among the individual medical specialties, proportions of choices remain fairly constant over the years except for the substantial rise in choices for geriatrics, which appears to level off after about eight or nine years.

Table 10.1 Medicine: percentages of first choices of career (tied or untied, corrected for ties), see Parkhouse and Ellin 1990c

		Years after qualifying						
Specialty	*Year of qualifying*	*1*	*3*	*5*	*7*	*9*	*11*	*13*
General medicine	1974	18.4	8.5	5.4	4.2	3.8	4.2	4.0
	1977	16.2	7.5	4.8	3.5	3.6		
Cardiology	1974	0.7	0.4	0.7	0.7	0.6	0.5	0.6
	1977	0.7	0.6	0.7	0.6	0.5		
Clinical pharmacology	1974	0.4	0.2	0.2	0.4	0.3	0.3	0.3
	1977	0.1	0.1	0.1	–	0.1		
Communicable diseases	1974	–	–	0.1	0.2	0.2	0.3	0.2
	1977	0.2	0.2	0.2	0.2	0.2		
Dermatology	1974	0.8	1.1	1.0	0.9	0.9	0.9	0.8
	1977	0.6	1.1	1.1	1.1	1.1		
Endocrinology	1974	0.1	0.4	0.1	0.5	0.3	0.1	0.1
	1977	0.2	0.3	0.4	0.4	0.4		
Gastroenterology	1974	0.2	0.5	0.3	0.3	0.2	0.3	0.4
	1977	0.2	0.1	0.1	0.1	0.1		
Genito-urinary medicine	1974	–	0.2	0.1	0.2	0.3	0.3	0.3
	1977	–	–	–	0.1	0.2		
Geriatrics	1974	0.3	0.4	0.8	0.9	1.1	1.1	1.2
	1977	0.3	0.8	0.6	0.8	1.1		
Haematology	1974	1.1	0.7	1.3	1.5	1.3	1.5	1.3
	1977	0.9	1.3	1.3	1.4	1.3		

Table 10.1 continued

Specialty	Year of qualifying	Years after qualifying						
		1	*3*	*5*	*7*	*9*	*11*	*13*
Medical genetics	1974	0.2	0.2	0.2	0.1	0.2	0.2	0.2
	1977	–	–	0.1	0.1	0.2		
Nephrology	1974	0.1	0.4	0.2	0.3	0.2	0.1	0.2
	1977	0.1	0.1	0.2	0.2	0.2		
Neurology	1974	0.7	1.5	0.9	0.8	0.8	0.9	0.9
	1977	0.5	0.6	0.5	0.5	0.5		
Rheumatology	1974	0.2	0.5	0.7	0.7	0.6	0.7	0.9
	1977	0.2	0.7	0.4	0.5	0.6		
Thoracic medicine	1974	0.1	0.3	0.5	0.6	0.6	0.4	0.2
	1977	0.2	0.5	1.0	0.8	0.5		
Tropical medicine	1974	0.2	0.3	0.1	–	–	–	0.1
	1977	0.3	0.2	0.1	0.2	0.2		
Other medicine	1974	0.2	0.4	0.3	0.3	0.6	0.5	0.5
	1977	0.4	0.6	0.4	0.4	0.6		
Medicine total	1974	23.6	15.8	12.8	12.6	12.0	12.3	12.2
	1977	21.0	14.9	12.1	11.0	11.3		

Table 10.2 Medical posts held by 1974 qualifiers in April 1983

Specialty	*SHO*	*Reg.*	*SR*	*Cons.*	*Academic*	*Clinical asst, etc. (GP)*[a]	*Other*[b]	*Total*
General medicine	–	4	38	7	22	9 (9)	18	98
Cardiology	–	–	3	–	8	3 (3)	4	18
Clinical pharmacology	–	–	–	–	7	–	1	8
Communicable diseases	–	–	1	–	1	–	1	3
Dermatology	–	5	5	3	3	8 (7)	–	24
Endocrinology	–	–	–	–	3	6 (6)[c]	1	10
Gastroenterology	–	–	–	–	4	7 (7)	2	13
Genito-urinary medicine	–	–	2	3	1	4 (1)	–	10
Geriatrics	–	3	7	7	1	15 (13)[d]	3	36
Haematology	1	2	10	7	7	2 (1)	1	30
Medical genetics	–	–	–	1	–	1 (0)	–	2
Nephrology	–	–	2	–	3	–	1	6
Neurology	–	6	4	1	4	3 (2)	2	20
Rheumatology	–	2	6	–	2	6 (5)	1	17
Thoracic medicine	–	2	1	2	3	3 (3)	1	12
Tropical medicine	–	–	–	–	1	–	–	1
Other medicine	–	1	–	–	2	12 (9)[e]	7	22
Medicine total	1	25	79	31	72	79 (66)	43	330

Notes: a Number of general practitioners in parentheses (including three in general medicine and one in cardiology abroad)
b Including posts abroad and in the Armed Forces
c Including five clinical assistants in diabetes
d Including one clinical assistant in geriatrics and orthopaedics
e Including six clinical assistants and two different medical specialties

CAREER PROGRESS

Tables 10.2 and 10.3 show the medical posts held by 1974 and 1977 qualifiers at comparable times after qualifying — in April of the ninth year after leaving medical school, which is the latest time for which we have comparable data. Of the 1974 qualifiers working in medicine, 9.4 per cent had achieved consultant status, compared to 7.6 per cent of 1977 qualifiers after an equivalent period of time. This difference is reflected in the fact that 32.1 per cent of 1977 qualifiers were in the senior registrar grade, compared to only 23.9 per cent of 1974 qualifiers. Substantial numbers of people from both years were in academic posts, and these include a variety of appointments variously described as research assistant, research associate, research registrar, etc. Also, substantial numbers of those working in medicine occupied clinical assistantships or similar types of appointments — 20.0 per cent from the two years combined, and 76.3 per cent of these doctors were combining their medical commitment with general practice.

Table 10.4 shows the latest information available from our data — the medical posts held by 1974 qualifiers thirteen years after leaving medical school. As would be expected, the numbers having achieved consultant status show a large rise — to 33.8 per cent. The numbers occupying clinical assistantships have also risen, however, to 29.9 per cent of those working in medicine, although the number of general practitioners in this group, according to our information, was only three more than four years previously. Fewer academic post were held, and this is in accordance with the transient nature of many of these appointments and the fact that they tend to be occupied en route to a senior registrarship or consultant appointment.

Table 10.5 shows the range and variety of medical experience obtained abroad by 1974 and 1977 qualifiers. Of all respondents from the two years, 6.2 per cent had held medical appointments overseas, the majority of these being in general medicine, and the next more popular specialty being cardiology. Of those who had been abroad, 29.3 per cent had spent a total of more than two years overseas and 9.9 per cent had held four or more jobs abroad.

SENIOR REGISTRARS AND CONSULTANTS IN MEDICINE

Table 10.6 shows the approximate time taken to achieve a substantive (i.e. non-locum) senior registrar or consultant post

Table 10.5 Medical experience abroad (1974 and 1977 qualifiers combined)

Specialty	*No.*	*(%) of respondents*	*No. of jobs held abroad*					*Duration of jobs held abroad (mths)*				
			1	*2*	*3*	*4*	*4+*	*0-6*	*6-12*	*12-24*	*24+*	*?*
General medicine	220	(4.2)	149	45	16	8	2	49	98	96	48	38
Cardiology	27	(0.5)	19	5	1	–	2	7	10	8	9	10
Clinical pharmacology	8	(0.2)	6	1	1	–	–	–	1	4	4	2
Communicable diseases	9	(0.2)	9	–	–	–	–	–	2	4	1	2
Dermatology	8	(0.2)	6	2	–	–	–	2	3	3	–	2
Endocrinology	19	(0.4)	15	2	1	1	–	2	4	12	2	6
Gastroenterology	14	(0.3)	11	2	1	–	–	3	2	5	4	4
Genito-urinary medicine	2	–	1	1	–	–	–	2	1	–	–	–
Geriatrics	10	(0.2)	9	1	–	–	–	5	–	3	–	3
Haematology	10	(0.2)	6	3	–	–	1	1	3	5	5	3
Medical genetics	6	(0.1)	4	2	–	–	–	–	–	3	2	3
Nephrology	10	(0.2)	8	1	1	–	–	5	3	3	1	1
Neurology	13	(0.2)	12	–	1	–	–	6	2	2	2	3
Rheumatology	20	(0.4)	18	2	–	–	–	6	6	5	3	2
Thoracic medicine	16	(0.3)	12	2	1	1	–	5	6	7	3	2
Tropical medicine	6	(0.1)	4	2	–	–	–	–	1	4	3	–
Other medicine	11	(0.2)	10	1	–	–	–	1	3	2	4	2
GP/Medicine	8	(0.2)	8	–	–	–	–	1	–	1	4	2
Medicine total	324	(6.2)	203	63	26	13	19	95	145	167	95	85

Table 10.5 continued

Specialty	*Nos of jobs held by country abroad*								*Nos. of academic posts abroad*
	EC	*Other Europe*	*Australia*	*New Zealand*	*Canada*	*USA*	*Other*	*Various*	
General medicine	18	9	50	53	38	38	122	1	11
Cardiology	1	–	10	12	2	17	2	–	7
Clinical pharmacology	–	1	3	3	–	4	–	–	6
Communicable diseases	–	–	1	1	–	6	1	–	2
Dermatology	2	–	1	1	–	4	2	–	3
Endocrinology	2	–	4	3	2	15	–	–	5
Gastroenterology	–	–	–	4	4	9	1	–	6
Genito-urinary medicine	–	–	–	–	–	–	3	–	–
Geriatrics	1	–	4	4	2	–	–	–	1
Haematology	–	–	7	2	1	5	2	–	2
Medical genetics	–	–	2	–	1	5	–	–	2
Nephrology	–	–	–	7	1	1	4	–	–
Neurology	–	–	1	6	1	6	1	–	2
Rheumatology	–	1	3	7	3	6	2	–	5
Thoracic medicine	–	–	1	8	10	2	2	–	1
Tropical medicine	1	–	–	–	1	–	5	1	3
Other medicine	–	2	1	1	1	4	2	1	2
GP/Medicine	–	–	1	–	2	–	5	–	–
Medicine total	25	13	89	112	69	122	154	3	58

Table 10.6 Years taken to achieve first non-locum senior registrar and consultant posts in medical disciplines, see Parkhouse and Ellin 1990c

	Senior registrar						*Consultant*					
	1974 qualifiers			*1977 qualifiers*			*1974 qualifiers*			*1977 qualifiers*		
Specialty	*no.*	*range*	*mean*	*no.*	*range*	*mean*	*no.*	*range*	*mean*	*no.*	*range*	*mean*
General medicine	60	4-12	7.8	49	5-9	7.1	42	7-13	10.6	9	8-10	8.7
Cardiology	3	8-10	9.0	4	5-9	7.0	1	11	–	–	–	–
Clinical pharmacology	3	5-6	5.3	2	5-9	7.0	–	–	–	–	–	–
Communicable diseases	2	5-8	6.5	1	6	–	1	9	–	–	–	–
Dermatology	11	5-11	7.2	14	4-8	6.2	8	8-12	9.8	4	7-9	8.3
Endocrinology	–	–	–	3	5-8	6.3	–	–	–	–	–	–
Gastroenterology	2	4-9	6.5	–	–	–	2	11-12	11.5	–	–	–
Genito-urinary medicine	6	4-7	5.5	1	5	–	5	6-9	8.2	1	9	–
Geriatrics	18	4-12	6.9	20	4-9	6.7	15	6-13	8.9	10	7-9	8.1
Haematology	20	4-12	6.6	27	4-9	6.1	16	8-13	9.5	4	8-9	8.8
Medical genetics	1	4	–	1	5	–	2	7-12	9.5	1	7	–
Nephrology	1	3	–	4	5-7	6.0	–	–	–	1	9	–
Neurology	11	6-11	8-9	4	6-9	7.3	4	8-13	10.8	–	–	–
Rheumatology	9	5-10	6.6	6	4-9	7.0	7	11-13	11.6	1	10	–
Thoracic medicine	2	6	6.0	5	6-9	8.2	3	7-10	8.3	–	–	–
Tropical medicine	–	–	–	–	–	–	–	–	–	–	–	–
Other medicine[a]	–	–	–	–	–	–	1	11	–	1	5	–
Medicine total	149	3-12	7.3	141	4-9	6.7	107	6-13	10.0	32	5-10	8.3
All hospital specialties	579	3-13	7.4	593	3-10	6.5	407	6-13	10.1	190	5-10	8.3

Note: a Terminal care

for the first time. Although most respondents gave the month and year of obtaining the relevant posts, we did not, in many cases, know the exact month of qualifying from medical school. The numbers of years shown in the table are therefore derived by subtracting the year of qualification from the year of the first substantive appointment in the grade concerned. The figures in Table 10.6 exclude holders of academic and honorary posts at senior registrar or consultant level.

An important point to note about this table, and the comparable tables in the following chapters relating to other individual specialties, is that 1977 qualifiers had been followed for only nine years, while 1974 qualifiers had been followed for thirteen years. Among the 1977 qualifiers, therefore, those who had become senior registrars by the time they last replied to us, and even more so those who had become consultants, tended to be the fast-moving 'high-fliers' within their various specialties. The fact that for this reason the average times for the two cohorts are not strictly comparable is confirmed by the evidence from Tables 10.2 and 10.3 that, as a whole, the 1977 qualifiers were moving less rapidly towards consultant appointments than the 1974 qualifiers at nine years after leaving medical school.

Table 10.6 shows that for medicine as a whole the rate of progress towards senior registrar and consultant appointments was very much the same as the average for all hospital specialties, as derived from our data. In some medical specialties, such as neurology, progress was slower than average.

Table 10.7 shows that 79.0 per cent of those doctors who had achieved senior registrar or consultant status in general medicine had given this specialty as their specific first choice of career one and/or three years after qualifying. Likewise, almost 70 per cent of those becoming senior registrars or consultants in neurology had done so. By contrast, considerably fewer than half of the doctors who became senior registrars or consultants in the majority of medical specialties had named the specific discipline as a career choice soon after leaving medical school — only 16.3 per cent of those in geriatrics. This fits with the changes in choice over the years shown in Table 10.1, and reveals once more the prevailing lack of opportunity for finding out about many branches of medical work during the undergraduate course and soon after qualifying. It also reflects the reappraisal of career opportunities in general medicine, as compared to some of the medical specialties, and the awakening of interest in the specific aspects of medical work as more clinical experience is gained. A summary of the picture of progress in relation to career choice, for medicine as a whole, is given in Table 10.8. Some idea of the

Table 10.7 Achievement in relation to career choice in medicine (1974 and 1977 qualifiers combined)

Specialty	*No. becoming non-locum SR and/or consultant*	*No. choosing specific discipline 1 and/or 3 years after qualifying*	*No. not choosing specific discipline 1 and/or 3 years after qualifying*	*Invalid due to absent replies*
General medicine	119	94	13	12
Cardiology	7	1	5	1
Clinical pharmacology	6	1	3	2
Communicable diseases	4	1	3	–
Dermatology	29	13	6	10
Endocrinology	3	–	2	1
Gastroenterology	2	1	–	1
Genito-urinary medicine	8	2	4	2
Geriatrics	43	7	29	7
Haematology	52	28	7	17
Medical genetics	3	1	2	–
Nephrology	5	2	1	2
Neurology	16	11	2	3
Rheumatology	15	6	5	4
Thoracic medicine	8	2	2	4
Tropical medicine	–	–	–	–
Other medicine	3	1	2	–
Medicine total	323	171	86	66

Table 10.8 Progress in relation to career choice: all medical disciplines combined

Year of qualifying	*No. becoming non-locum SR and/or consultant in a medical discipline*	*No. (%) choosing a specific discipline 1 and/or 3 years after qualifying*		*Total no. choosing a medical discipline 1 and/or 3 years after qualifying*	*No. (%) choosing medicine 1 and/or 3 years after qualifying who had not become a non-locum SR and/or consultant in a medical discipline*	
1974	175	89	(50.9)	516	427	(82.8)
1977	148	82	(55.4)	681	599	(88.0)
1974 and 1977 combined	323	171	(52.9)	1,197	1,026	(85.7)

Table 10.9 Experience obtained before becoming consultants in a medical discipline (1974 and 1977 qualifiers combined), see Parkhouse and Ellin 1990c

Specialty	*No. of respondents*	*General medicine (yrs)*				*Other medical specialties*	*Other hospital specialties*	*GP*	*Academic*	*Basic sciences*	*Other incl. abroad*	*SR equivalent*
		0-1	*1-2*	*2+*	*?*[a]							
General medicine	52	–	–	–	–	46	17	2	34	3	12	4
Cardiology	1	–	–	–	1	–	–	–	1	–	–	–
Clinical pharmacology	–	–	–	–	–	–	–	–	–	–	–	–
Communicable diseases	1	–	1	–	–	1	–	–	–	–	1	–
Dermatology	12	1	6	3	2 (1)	5	3	–	4	–	2	3
Endocrinology	–	–	–	–	–	–	–	–	–	–	–	–
Gastroenterology	2	–	–	2	–	2	–	–	1	–	1	–
Genito-urinary medicine	6	–	1	1	4 (4)	3	5	3	3	1	1	1
Geriatrics	25	–	4	19	2	16	12	4	6	1	4	4
Haematology	20	4	7	5	4 (4)	6	9	–	8	–	1	4
Medical genetics	3	–	1	–	2 (2)	1	3	1	2	–	1	1
Nephrology	1	–	–	1	–	–	–	–	1	–	–	–
Neurology	4	–	3	1	–	3	2	–	4	1	–	1
Rheumatology	8	–	3	5	–	4	5	–	5	1	1	–
Thoracic medicine	2	–	–	2	–	–	–	–	1	–	–	–
Tropical medicine	–	–	–	–	–	–	–	–	–	–	–	–
Other medicine	2	1	–	–	1	–	2	–	–	–	1	2
Medicine total	139	6	26	39	16(11)	87	58	10	70	7	25	20

Note: a Numbers in parentheses are those not recording any post–registration experience specifically in general medicine

size of the career problem is given by the fact that of the 1977 qualifiers who gave medicine as their first choice of career one and/or three years after qualifying, there were 88 per cent who had not achieved senior registrar or consultant status in a medical discipline nine years after leaving medical school.

Table 10.9 gives a breakdown of the variety of experience obtained on the way to becoming a consultant in a medical discipline. Outside general medicine and the medical specialties, this appears to be quite limited: only ten people altogether, from both cohorts, had had experience in general practice, and only seven in the basic sciences. This no doubt indicates that the generality of 'medicine' is a very wide field, within which most doctors feel that they can obtain as much variety of relevant experience as they need. A number of those who had become consultants had not, according to our records, held regular NHS senior registrar posts, but had obtained equivalent experience in other ways, including appointments abroad.

Taking 1974 and 1977 qualifiers together, 45.1 per cent of those who had become senior registrars in medicine held their senior registrarship in the region of their medical school and 31.4 per cent of those who had become consultants in medicine held their consultant posts in the region of their medical school. Taking both cohorts, 20.7 per cent had held both senior registrar and consultant posts in the region of their medical school, and 40.5 per cent had been senior registrars and consultants in the same region, regardless of which region it was. The inclusion of Belfast graduates in the 1977 survey affects these figures, since fourteen out of fourteen Belfast graduates had become senior registrars in medicine in Northern Ireland and four out of four had become consultants in medicine in Northern Ireland. Even when these figures are excluded from the 1977 data, however, the percentage who had become senior registrars in the region of their medical school was 45.6 among 1977 qualifiers, compared to 40.2 per cent among 1974 qualifiers. Similarly the percentage who had become consultants in their medical school region was 34.5 among 1977 qualifiers, compared to only 27.9 per cent among 1974 qualifiers.

Among the doctors who had been senior registrars in medicine there were twelve 1974 qualifiers and seven 1977 qualifiers who were known to have worked part-time at some stage. Of these nineteen respondents, seventeen were women. At their latest replies to us, five were working in dermatology, all of whom were 1974 qualifiers; four were in haematology, three being 1974 qualifiers; eight others were each in a different branch of medicine; one was in general practice and one was

Table 10.10 Respondents in 1987 who had held, at any time, substantive registrar posts in general medicine: posts held in 1987 (1974 qualifiers), see Parkhouse and Ellin 1990c

Specialty	*No. of respondents*	*Grade*						*Location*	
		Reg.	*SR*	*Cons.*	*Academic*	*Principal*	*Other*	*UK*	*Abroad*
General medicine	65	2	15	39	7	–	2	63	2
Cardiology	4	–	–	1	2	–	1	4	–
Clinical pharmacology	3	–	–	–	3	–	–	3	–
Communicable diseases	1	–	–	–	1	–	–	1	–
Dermatology	10	–	2	4	1	–	3	10	–
Endocrinology	1	–	–	–	–	–	1	–	1
Gastroenterology	2	–	–	1	–	–	1	1	1
Genito-urinary medicine	1	–	–	–	1	–	–	1	–
Geriatrics	17	–	–	14	2	–	1	16	1
Haematology	9	–	2	5	2	–	–	9	–
Nephrology	–	–	–	–	–	–	–	–	–
Neurology	8	–	1	3	4	–	–	7	1
Rheumatology	10	–	–	6	3	–	1	9	1
Thoracic medicine	2	–	–	2	–	–	–	2	–
Tropical medicine	1	–	–	–	1	–	–	1	–
Other medicine	3	–	–	1	1	–	1	3	–
GP/medicine	9	–	–	–	–	8	1	8	1
Accident and emergency	1	–	–	1	–	–	–	1	–
Anaesthetics	4	–	1	2	–	–	1	3	1
Obstetrics and gynaecology	2	–	–	–	1	–	1	2	–

Table 10.10 continued

Specialty	*No. of respondents*	*Grade*						*Location*	
		Reg.	*SR*	*Cons.*	*Academic*	*Principal*	*Other*	*UK*	*Abroad*
Ophthalmology	1	–	–	1	–	–	–	1	–
Paediatrics	2	–	–	2	–	–	–	2	–
Pathology	2	–	1	–	–	–	1	1	1
Psychiatry	4	1	–	2	1	–	–	4	–
Radiology	7	–	1	5	1	–	–	6	1
Radiotherapy	3	–	–	1	1	–	1	2	1
General practice	43	–	–	–	–	36	7	42	1
Community medicine	4	–	–	–	–	–	4	3	1
Other medical work	5	–	–	–	–	–	5	5	–
Not working	2	–	–	–	–	–	2	1	–
Total	226	3	23	90	32	44	34	211	14

unemployed. Thirteen were currently part-time senior registrars and two were full-time senior registrars, one after doing part-time sessional work in genito-urinary medicine and one with concurrent locum registrar sessions. One was a part-time consultant following a part-time senior registrarship; one was a part-time clinical assistant; one had become a general practice trainee and one, previously working in haematology, was unemployed as a result of moving with her husband.

Five respondents specifically mentioned maternity and family commitments as a reason for breaks in employment and part-time work; the same could be inferred in some other cases. Five respondents mentioned moves with a husband and in one case this problem was complicated by ill-health. Two respondents mentioned having used the Women Doctors' Retainer Scheme.

WHAT HAPPENS TO MEDICAL REGISTRARS?

The main difficulty in career progression, in the highly competitive specialties which show a large imbalance between the numbers of junior and senior posts, is in getting from the registrar to the senior registrar grade. Little follow-up information is available about what actually happens to all the doctors who have been registrars in medicine. Such an analysis is complicated by the fact that many registrar posts in 'general medicine' involve rotation through a variety of medical disciplines such as thoracic medicine, cardiology, neurology, etc. On the other hand, other registrar posts in neurology, and almost all of those in dermatology, are regarded as specific training posts for their own specialty. Only interim information is available from our studies to date, but Table 10.10 gives an analysis of the jobs held by 1974 qualifiers who responded to us in 1987 and who had, at any time, held substantive registrar posts in general medicine. Thirty-nine respondents (17.3 per cent) were consultants in general medicine, and thirty-seven (16.4 per cent) were consultants in other medical specialties. Fourteen respondents (6.2 per cent) had become consultants in hospital specialties outside medicine, and forty-four (19.5 per cent) were principals in general practice. Only fourteen (6.2 per cent) were working abroad, and only three were still registrars — two in general medicine and one in psychiatry.

11 Individual specialties

Surgery

The term 'surgery' is used to embrace all branches of surgical work, as listed in the tables; it includes ophthalmology and accident and emergency. The term 'general surgery' is used to include doctors who described their career choices or jobs as surgery, general surgery, academic surgery, and surgery or general surgery with an interest in a special field of surgical practice. Vascular surgery is included in general surgery; other kinds of surgical work, such as transplant surgery, head and neck surgical oncology, and specialized work not clearly described, are grouped together as 'other surgery'.

CAREER CHOICES

Table 11.1 shows the dramatic decline in choices for general surgery from over 10 per cent to less than 3 per cent after nine to eleven years, which applies to both 1974 and 1977 qualifiers. Most surgical specialties remained constant or increased in popularity during these years after qualifying and, although the numbers are small, ENT appeared more popular among 1977 qualifiers than among those of 1974.

Ophthalmology was by far the commonest surgical choice among women; in the pre-registration year 24.7 per cent of 1974 qualifiers choosing ophthalmology, and 25.4 per cent of 1977 qualifiers, were women. Nine years after qualifying these figures had risen to 40.9 and 30.3 per cent respectively. In accident and emergency, women 1977 qualifiers provided between 21 and 36 per cent of the first choices during the nine years after qualifying; but among 1974 qualifiers accident and emergency lost popularity among women doctors after the pre-registration year, except for a surge of interest seven years after qualifying (26.7 per cent of choices), while its popularity among men increased mainly beyond the seven-year period from qualifying.

Table 11.1 Surgery: percentages of first choices of career (tied or untied, corrected for ties)

Specialty	*Year of qualifying*	*Years after qualifying* 1	3	5	7	9	11	13
General surgery	1974	10.2	6.2	4.7	3.7	3.2	2.9	2.6
	1977	11.2	6.1	3.8	3.4	2.7		
Accident and emergency	1974	0.5	0.3	0.4	0.4	0.8	0.8	0.8
	1977	0.3	0.4	0.8	1.0	0.9		
ENT	1974	0.2	0.4	0.4	0.7	0.6	0.5	0.5
	1977	0.5	0.8	1.1	1.3	1.3		
Neurosurgery	1974	0.4	0.3	0.3	0.3	0.3	0.2	0.3
	1977	0.2	0.2	0.2	0.2	0.2		
Ophthalmology	1974	0.7	1.3	1.2	1.2	1.1	1.3	1.3
	1977	1.1	1.4	1.4	1.3	1.3		
Orthopaedics	1974	2.0	2.0	2.3	2.1	2.0	1.7	1.8
	1977	2.3	3.1	2.8	2.4	2.4		
Paediatric surgery	1974	0.3	0.1	0.2	0.2	0.1	0.1	0.1
	1977	0.1	0.2	0.2	0.1	0.2		
Plastic surgery	1974	0.4	0.4	0.3	0.4	0.6	0.6	0.5
	1977	0.5	0.4	0.4	0.4	0.3		
Cardiothoracic surgery	1974	0.5	0.2	0.5	0.5	0.6	0.6	0.4
	1977	0.3	0.2	0.3	0.4	0.3		

Table 11.1 continued

Specialty	*Year of qualifying*	*Years after qualifying*						
		1	*3*	*5*	*7*	*9*	*11*	*13*
Urology	1974	0.1	0.2	0.6	0.6	0.8	0.7	0.8
	1977	0.1	0.1	0.2	0.5	0.5		
Other surgery	1974	0.4	0.4	0.1	0.1	0.2	0.2	0.2
	1977	0.4	0.3	0.2	–	0.1		
Surgery total	1974	15.8	11.8	10.9	10.1	10.3	9.6	9.4
	1977	17.0	13.2	11.4	11.0	10.2		

Table 11.2 Surgical posts held by 1974 qualifiers up to 1987

Specialty	*SHO*			*Registrar*			*SR*			*Consultant*			*Academic*			*Other/ unknown*			*No. holding one or more surgical posts (% of 2,272)*
	FT	*PT*	*Loc*	*FT*	*PT*	*Loc*	*FT*	*PT*	*Loc*	*FT*	*PT*	*Loc*	*FT*	*PT*	*Loc*	*FT*	*PT*	*Loc*	
General surgery	215	1	13	170	0	23	41	0	17	18	0	5	41	1	3	76	2	8	306(13.5%)
Accident & emergency	708	13	29	26	1	4	13	0	2	9	0	1	0	1	0	52	24	14	813(35.8%)
ENT	54	0	4	13	0	0	9	0	0	6	0	0	2	0	0	8	4	0	70 (3.1%)
Neurosurgery	34	0	3	23	0	2	7	0	0	5	0	0	0	0	0	5	0	0	60 (2.6%)
Ophthalmology	48	3	4	20	1	3	16	1	2	13	1	2	3	0	0	11	12	4	57 (2.5%)
Orthopaedics	114	0	8	73	0	7	30	0	6	15	0	2	15	0	1	31	4	2	182 (8.0%)
Paediatric surgery	19	0	1	19	0	0	1	0	0	0	0	0	0	0	0	2	0	0	41 (1.8%)
Plastic surgery	21	0	5	17	1	4	3	0	0	1	0	0	3	0	0	8	1	0	39 (1.7%)
Cardiothoracic surgery	25	0	1	46	1	2	8	0	1	4	0	0	3	0	0	9	0	1	72 (3.2%)
Urology	46	0	0	32	1	5	18	0	2	7	0	0	10	0	0	10	1	0	90 (4.0%)
Other surgery	11	0	2	10	0	1	1	0	2	0	0	0	6	0	0	8	0	1	39 (1.7%)
Surgery total	831	17	57	238	5	45	138	1	30	78	1	10	83	2	4	182	47	29	976(43.0%)

Table 11.3 Surgical posts held by 1977 qualifiers up to 1986

Specialty	*SHO*			*Registrar*			*SR*			*Consultant*			*Academic*			*Other/ unknown*			*No. holding one or more surgical posts (% of 2,988)*	
	FT	*PT*	*Loc*	*FT*	*PT*	*Loc*	*FT*	*PT*	*Loc*	*FT*	*PT*	*Loc*	*FT*	*PT*	*Loc*	*FT*	*PT*	*Loc*		
General surgery	298	2	24	204	0	28	12	0	6	1	0	0	50	0	1	81	0	5	378	12.7%
Accident & emergency	1,094	38	72	37	1	5	11	0	0	4	0	1	0	0	0	52	38	11	1,215	40.7%
ENT	128	0	12	32	0	6	18	1	4	4	0	0	5	0	0	16	4	1	150	5.0%
Neurosurgery	56	1	8	27	0	2	2	0	0	0	0	0	1	0	0	1	0	0	90	3.0%
Ophthalmology	77	1	9	29	1	7	17	0	3	9	0	1	5	0	0	26	14	2	86	2.9%
Orthopaedics	188	1	17	103	1	13	22	0	4	1	0	0	12	0	0	23	4	2	273	9.1%
Paediatric surgery	26	0	0	19	0	0	1	0	0	0	0	0	1	0	0	2	0	0	43	1.4%
Plastic surgery	29	3	8	24	2	3	1	0	1	0	0	0	3	0	0	3	0	0	60	2.0%
Cardiothoracic surgery	56	0	7	47	0	1	6	0	3	0	0	0	2	0	1	3	0	1	106	3.5%
Urology	57	0	5	38	0	6	3	0	0	0	0	0	4	0	0	10	0	0	99	3.3%
Other surgery	29	1	4	14	0	2	1	0	0	0	0	0	2	0	0	6	1	0	57	1.9%
Surgery total	1,291	43	143	317	5	62	92	1	21	19	0	2	85	0	2	170	61	21	1,423	47.6%

SURGICAL EXPERIENCE

Tables 11.2 and 11.3 show the spread of post-registration surgical experience among 1977 qualifiers by the time they had been qualified nine years, and among 1974 qualifiers up to thirteen years after qualifying. These indications will be underestimates of the true amount of surgical experience among all qualifiers, since the data include those who did not respond to our questionnaires in 1986 and 1987 respectively, but who had responded on one or more previous occasions.

The figures for 1974 qualifiers (Table 11.2) show that by thirteen years after leaving medical school, and not including the pre-registration year, 43.0 per cent of respondents were known to have had surgical experience of some kind; the commonest type of work was in accident and emergency (35.8 per cent of respondents), nearly always as a full-time SHO, and the next commonest experience was general surgery (13.5 per cent of respondents). Most 1974 qualifiers were not involved in organized vocational training for general practice; only 3.1 per cent had gained any experience of ENT surgery and 2.5 per cent of ophthalmology — fewer than the number with experience of cardiothoracic surgery.

Table 11.3 shows that among 1977 qualifiers, nine years after leaving medical school 47.6 per cent of respondents had obtained some post-registration surgical experience — a higher proportion than was the case among 1974 qualifiers, even when reviewed thirteen years after leaving medical school (Table 11.2); this was largely due to increased involvement with accident and emergency (40.7 per cent of respondents) and ENT (5.0 per cent). This may be attributable, in part, to a growing emphasis on vocational training for general practice, although the higher exposure to ENT carried through to registrar and senior registrar levels.

CAREER PROGRESS

Tables 11.4 and 11.5 show the numbers of 1974 and 1977 qualifiers working in surgery at comparable times, nine years after qualifying. Rates of progress were similar, 4.0-4.7 per cent having become consultants although proportionately more of the 1974 qualifiers than those of 1977 were working as clinical assistants. The relatively high popularity of ENT surgery and ophthalmology among 1977 qualifiers was confirmed by the jobs held, and ophthalmology had the highest number of consultants of any branch of surgery, after nine years, from both cohorts.

Table 11.4 Surgical posts held by 1974 qualifiers in April 1983

Specialty	*SHO*	*Reg.*	*SR*	*Cons.*	*Academic*	*Clinical asst, etc.*	*(GP)*[a]	*Other*[b]	*Total*
General surgery	1	15	20	1	15	2	(2)	19	73
Accident & emergency	3	2	6	1	0	21	(16)	3	36
ENT	1	2	5	2	1	6	(5)	1	18
Neurosurgery	0	2	4	1	0	0		0	7
Ophthalmology	1	2	7	3	3	6	(1)[c]	3	25
Orthopaedics	1	13	15	0	7	6	(6)	7	49
Paediatric surgery	0	1	0	0	0	0		0	1
Plastic surgery	0	4	3	0	0	0		4	11
Cardiothoracic surgery	0	6	5	1	0	0		1	13
Urology	0	2	8	1	2	0		1	14
Other surgery	0	0	1	0	2	0		1	4
Surgery total	7	49	74	10	30	41	(30)	40	251

Notes: a Number of general practitioners in parentheses
b Including posts held abroad and in the Armed Forces
c Also clinical assistant in accident and emergency

Table 11.5 Surgical posts held by 1977 qualifiers in April 1986

Specialty	*SHO*	*Reg.*	*SR*	*Cons.*	*Academic*	*Clinical asst, etc. (GP)*[a]	*Other*[b]	*Total*
General surgery	1	17	11	0	23	1 (1)[c]	11	64
Accident & emergency	5	4	5	3	0	15 (12)[d]	6	38
ENT	1	3	19	1	1	4 (4)	4	33
Neurosurgery	1	3	2	0	0	0	1	7
Ophthalmology	0	3	7	9	2	7 (2)	5	33
Orthopaedics	1	21	19	0	9	5 (4)[e]	7	62
Paediatric surgery	1	3	1	0	0	0	0	5
Plastic surgery	3	5	0	0	1	1 (0)	0	10
Cardiothoracic surgery	0	3	4	0	1	0	1	9
Urology	0	5	3	0	2	0	2	12
Other surgery	1	2	0	0	1	0	2	6
Surgery total	14	69	71	13	40	33 (23)	39	279

Notes: a Number of general practitioners in parentheses
b Including posts held abroad and in the Armed Forces
c GP surgeon in the USA
d Including one GP/emergency medicine in Canada
e Including one also clinical assistant in accident and emergency

Table 11.6 Surgical posts held by 1974 qualifiers in 1987

Specialty	*SHO*	*Reg.*	*SR*	*Cons.*	*Academic*	*Clinical asst, etc. (GP)*[a]	*Other*[b]	*Total*
General surgery	0	4	23	18	8	5 (5)[c]	6	64
Accident & emergency	1	0	3	9	0	21 (17)	3	37
ENT	0	0	1	6	1	4 (4)	1	13
Neurosurgery	0	1	1	5	0	0	0	7
Ophthalmology	0	1	3	14	0	4 (o)	3 [d]	25
Orthopaedics	0	1	12	15	2	8 (8)[e]	5	43
Paediatric surgery	0	1	0	0	0	0	0	1
Plastic surgery	0	4	1	1	0	0	5 [f]	11
Cardiothoracic surgery	0	0	2	4	0	0	2	8
Urology	0	0	6	7	1	0	0	14
Other surgery	0	0	1	0	1	0	1	3
Surgery total	1	12	53	79	13	42 (34)	26	226

Notes: a Number of general practitioners in parentheses
b Including posts held abroad and in the Armed Forces
c Including one GP/surgeon in Canada
d Including one associate specialist
e Including one clinical assistant in spinal injuries
f Including one part-time private practitioner in cosmetic surgery

Table 11.7 Surgical experience abroad (1974 and 1977 qualifiers combined)

Specialty	*No.*	*(%) of respondents*	*No. of jobs held abroad*					*Duration of jobs held abroad (mths)*				
			1	*2*	*3*	*4*	*4+*	*0-6*	*6-12*	*12-24*	*24+*	*?*
General surgery	117	(2.2)	88	16	9	1	3	26	48	52	20	27
Accident & emergency	79	(1.5)	67	10	1	1	–	33	31	14	6	10
ENT	22	(0.4)	19	1	1	–	1	13	4	4	5	5
Neurosurgery	5	(0.1)	4	–	1	–	–	3	1	3	–	–
Ophthalmology	17	(0.3)	13	3	1	–	–	5	5	5	3	4
Orthopaedics	46	(0.9)	36	4	3	1	2	8	15	25	7	11
Paediatric surgery	4	(0.1)	3	1	–	–	–	–	4	–	1	–
Plastic surgery	9	(0.2)	6	3	–	–	–	2	3	1	2	4
Cardiothoracic surgery	12	(0.2)	10	2	–	–	–	3	4	3	1	3
Urology	7	(0.1)	6	1	–	–	–	2	3	1	–	2
Other surgery	8	(0.2)	7	1	–	–	–	1	4	2	–	2
GP/surgery	10	(0.2)	10	–	–	–	–	2	–	–	2	6
Surgery total	266	(5.1)	180	46	19	10	11	98	122	110	47	74

Table 11.7 continued

Specialty	*Nos of jobs held by country abroad*								*Nos. of academic posts abroad*
	EC	*Other Europe*	*Australia*	*New Zealand*	*Canada*	*USA*	*Other*	*Various*	
General surgery	10	11	20	32	9	21	67	3	7
Accident & emergency	6	1	16	16	8	8	39	–	1
ENT	2	7	1	6	2	5	8	–	2
Neurosurgery	–	1	1	–	1	1	3	–	–
Ophthalmology	2	–	3	4	3	3	7	–	–
Orthopaedics	6	3	8	9	21	10	9	–	4
Paediatric surgery	–	–	2	2	–	–	1	–	–
Plastic surgery	–	–	3	1	1	4	3	–	2
Cardiothoracic surgery	–	–	–	2	1	3	8	–	1
Urology	–	1	–	3	–	3	1	–	1
Other surgery	1	–	–	3	3	–	2	–	1
GP/surgery	–	–	2	1	5	–	1	1	–
Surgery total	27	24	56	79	54	58	149	4	19

Table 11.8 Years taken to achieve first non–locum senior registrar and consultant posts in surgical disciplines

	Senior registrar						*Consultant*					
	1974 qualifiers			*1977 qualifiers*			*1974 qualifiers*			*1977 qualifiers*		
Specialty	*no.*	*range*	*mean*	*no.*	*range*	*mean*	*no.*	*range*	*mean*	*no.*	*range*	*mean*
General surgery	38	5-13	9.1	9	5-9	7.7	18	9-13	11.3	1	–	9.0
Accident & emergency	12	5-10	8.1	11	4-9	6.1	9	9-12	10.7	4	6-9	7.5
ENT	9	5-9	6.6	19	5-9	6.5	6	8-11	9.7	4	9-10	9.3
Neurosurgery	5	6-10	7.6	1	–	7.0	5	9-12	10.8	–	–	–
Ophthalmology	16	5-12	7.0	16	4-8	5.8	14	7-13	10.0	9	7-9	8.0
Orthopaedics	29	5-13	8.7	22	6-9	8.0	15	10-13	11.8	–	–	–
Paediatric surgery	1	–	11.0	1	–	8.0	–	–	–	–	–	–
Plastic surgery	3	8-9	8.7	–	–	–	1	–	11.0	–	–	–
Cardiothoracic surgery	6	8-10	8.3	6	7-9	7.8	4	8-12	10.3	–	–	–
Urology	14	6-12	9.5	3	8-9	8.3	6	10-13	11.5	–	–	–
Other surgery	–	–	–	1	–	7.0	–	–	–	–	–	–
Surgery total	133	5-13	8.5	89	4-9	7.0	78	7-13	10.9	18	7-10	8.2
All hospital specialties	579	3-13	7.4	593	3-10	6.5	407	6-13	10.1	190	5-10	8.3

Table 11.9 Achievement in relation to career choice in surgery (1974 and 1977 qualifiers combined)

Specialty	*No. becoming non-locum SR and/or consultant*	*No. choosing specific discipline 1 and/or 3 years after qualifying*	*No. not choosing specific discipline 1 and/or 3 years after qualifying*	*Invalid due to absent replies*
General surgery	55	47	2	6
Accident & emergency	24	2	15	7
ENT	28	15	2	11
Neurosurgery	7	3	3	1
Ophthalmology	34	28	2	4
Orthopaedics	53	23	15	15
Paediatric surgery	2	0	2	0
Plastic surgery	3	2	1	0
Cardiothoracic surgery	13	2	6	5
Urology	18	1	11	6
Other surgery	1	0	0	1
Surgery total	238	123	59	56

Table 11.6 shows that four years later, the proportion of 1974 respondents in surgery who had achieved consultant status in the UK had risen from 4.0 to 35.0 per cent. The highest rate of consultant achievement among the larger surgical specialties was again in ophthalmology (56.0 per cent), compared to 34.9 per cent in orthopaedics, 28.1 per cent in general surgery and only 24.3 per cent in accident and emergency. In the smaller surgical specialties, five of the seven doctors working in neurosurgery were consultants and four of the eight in cardiothoracic surgery, compared to only one of eleven in plastic surgery.

Table 11.7 gives combined figures for 1974 and 1977 qualifiers showing surgical experience abroad. Of the 1974 respondents, 135 (5.9 per cent) had worked in surgery abroad at some time, compared to 131 of the 1977 respondents (4.4 per cent). Most experience abroad was obtained in the earlier years after qualification, so even allowing for the fact that 1974 qualifiers had been followed for longer, there is probably an indication of decline in overseas experience between the two cohorts. The pattern was also different: out of almost exactly equal total numbers working in surgery abroad, fifty-four 1977 qualifiers went to New Zealand compared to twenty-five 1974 qualifiers, while fewer 1977 qualifiers went to Australia (sixteen, compared to forty from 1974). Sixty-eight 1974 qualifiers went to the USA or Canada, but only forty-four 1977 qualifiers did so.

SENIOR REGISTRARS AND CONSULTANTS IN SURGERY

Table 11.8 shows times taken to achieve substantive senior registrar and consultant appointments. As in the case of medicine, to obtain a true mean for the time taken to achieve these grades it would be necessary to wait until the last person to obtain a post at the relevant level had done so. In this respect, the fact that 1974 qualifiers, having been followed for thirteen years, represented a wider range of different rates of advancement than 1977 qualifiers, is seen from the data.

Generally the most rapid progress was in ENT surgery, where the average times taken to become a senior registrar and a consultant were about six and a half years and nine and a half years respectively. However, the range around those means (and the 1977 figures) show that in accident and emergency and ophthalmology there were some qualifiers with an early career choice who progressed quickly, in comparison to the prevailing norm for surgery as a whole. That this norm was high is illustrated by the closest approach from the data to a true mean time for becoming a consultant, of almost eleven years, compared with just over ten years for 1974 qualifiers in all hospital specialties combined.

Table 11.9 shows that of the respondents who were known to have become senior registrars and/or consultants, 85.5 per cent of those in general surgery had given general surgery as their first choice of career one or three years after qualifying, or at both of those times. Comparable figures were 82.4 per cent of those in ophthalmology, 53.6 per cent in ENT, 43.4 per cent in orthopaedics and only 8.3 per cent in accident and emergency. Taking all surgical disciplines together (Table 11.10) just over half of those becoming senior registrars and/or consultants had made early career choices for their specific discipline. Among 1974 qualifiers, after thirteen years, 24.2 per cent of those whose first choice of career one and/or three years after qualifying was some kind of surgery had become surgical senior registrars or consultants; after nine years, only 9.0 per cent of comparable 1977 qualifiers had done so.

Table 11.11 shows the range of experience obtained after full registration and before becoming a surgical senior registrar, and shows also the amount of general surgical experience recorded by respondents who became senior registrars in other branches of surgery. Only 16.4 per cent of those becoming senior registrars in general surgery had obtained experience in any non-surgical hospital specialty, and none had worked in general practice. Among those becoming senior registrars in all surgical disciplines, from both 1974 and 1977 years of qualification, only 20.2 per cent had had non-surgical hospital experience since the pre-registration year and 5.0 per cent had worked in general practice; 37.8 per cent had held other kinds of medical posts, outside hospital or general practice, and this was most often part-time or full-time anatomy. Of those becoming senior registrars 85.3 per cent in ophthalmology and 42.9 per cent in ENT did not record any post-registration experience in general surgery. Four respondents (16.7 per cent) had become senior registrars in accident and emergency with the MRCP and with no recorded post-registration experience in general surgery.

On the way to becoming a surgical senior registrar, thirteen 1974 qualifiers (twelve men and one woman) and eleven 1977 qualifiers (ten men and one woman) were known to have held part-time posts. However, seventeen of these twenty-four part-time posts were held concurrently with other jobs, including one physiology and thirteen anatomy demonstratorships combined with SHO posts in accident and emergency or ophthalmology. Of

Table 11.10 Progress in relation to career choice: all surgical disciplines combined

Year of qualifying	*No. becoming non-locum SR and/or consultant in a surgical discipline*	*No. (%) choosing specific discipline 1 and/or 3 years after qualifying*	*Total no. choosing a surgical discipline 1 and/or 3 years after qualifying*	*No. (%) choosing surgery having not become a non-locum SR and/or consultant in a surgical discipline*
1974	147	77 (52.4)	318	241 (75.8)
1977	91	46 (50.5)	511	465 (91.0)
1974 and 1977 combined	238	123 (51.7)	829	706 (85.2)

Table 11.11 Experience obtained before becoming senior registrars in a surgical discipline (1974 and 1977 qualifiers combined)

Specialty	*No. of respondents*	*General surgery (yrs)*					*Other surgical specialties*	*Other hospital specialties*	*GP*	*Other medical*
		0	*0-1*	*1-2*	*2+*	*?*				
General surgery	55	–	–	–	–	–	53	9	–	25
Accident & emergency	24	4	1	11	8	–	15	11	3	7
ENT	28	12	5	9	2	–	25	1	2	11
Neurosurgery	7	–	1	5	1	–	6	2	–	2
Ophthalmology	34	29	3	2	–	–	20	9	3	10
Orthopaedics	53	–	2	29	17	5	53	11	3	22
Paediatric surgery	2	–	–	2	–	–	2	1	1	1
Plastic surgery	3	–	–	1	2	–	3	–	–	1
Cardiothoracic surgery	13	–	–	6	7	–	12	1	–	5
Urology	18	–	1	1	16	–	16	3	–	6
Other surgery	1	–	–	–	–	1	1	–	–	–
Surgery total	238	45	13	66	53	6	206	48	12	90

Table 11.12 Respondents in 1987 who had held, at any time, substantive registrar posts in general surgery: posts held in 1987 (1974 qualifiers)

	No. of	*Grade*						*Location*	
Specialty	*respondents*	*Reg.*	*SR*	*Cons.*	*Academic*	*Principal*	*Other*	*UK*	*Abroad*
General surgery	56	4	23	16	8	–	5	49	7
Accident & emergency	6	–	3	3	–	–	–	6	–
ENT	3	–	1	2	–	–	–	3	–
Neurosurgery	5	1	–	4	–	–	–	5	–
Ophthalmology	1	–	–	1	–	–	–	1	–
Orthopaedics	26	1	11	11	2	–	1	25	1
Plastic surgery	7	2	1	1	–	–	3	5	2
Cardiothoracic surgery	5	–	1	3	–	–	1	4	1
Urology	11	–	3	7	1	–	–	10	1
Other surgery	2	–	1	–	1	–	–	1	1
GP/surgery	3	–	–	–	–	2	1	2	1
General practice	8	–	–	–	–	7	1	8	–
Obstetrics & gynaecology	3	–	2	1	–	–	–	3	–
Radiology	5	2	3	–	–	–	–	5	–
Histopathology	1	–	–	1	–	–	–	1	–
Third World medicine	1	–	–	–	–	–	1	–	1
Other medical	2	–	–	–	1	–	1	–	2
Total	145	10	49	50	13	9	14	128	17

the seven instances in which respondents appeared to be genuinely working part-time, only one was a part-time senior registrarship, in ophthalmology, to accommodate domestic commitments in between full-time senior registrar and consultant appointments; the others comprised a part-time consultant post held by a man, and various clinical assistant and other posts, including part-time locums, held usually for short periods between full-time appointments.

Taking 1974 and 1977 qualifiers together, 238 respondents were known to have been substantive senior registrars and 97 were known to have been substantive consultants, in surgical disciplines. Of those with jobs in known locations, 46.0 per cent held their senior registrarships in the NHS region of their medical school (assuming any London medical school to be in any of the four Thames regions) and 36.1 per cent held their consultant posts in their medical school regions; 28.9 per cent had been both a senior registrar and a consultant in their medical school region. Altogether, 51.7 per cent held consultant posts in the region where they had been senior registrars. Among qualifiers from Scottish medical schools twenty-one out of forty (52.5 per cent) were known to have held surgical senior registrarships in England and Wales, and twelve of twenty-seven (44.4 per cent) held surgical consultant posts in England (none in Wales).

WHAT HAPPENS TO SURGICAL REGISTRARS?

Even more than in medicine, there are anxieties about a surplus of registrar posts in general surgery — posts which are increasingly often occupied by British graduates — in relation to senior registrar and consultant outlets. Obviously the question 'What happens to surgical registrars?' cannot be answered completely until enough time has elapsed for careers to run their full course, but an interim analysis based on our data is none the less interesting as far as it goes. In surgery, the individual disciplines tend to be more discrete than in medicine, so that although registrar posts in 'general surgery' often involve rotations to provide special experience, the great majority of registrar posts in neurosurgery, ENT surgery, ophthalmology, etc. are occupied by trainees in the disciplines concerned.

Table 11.12 shows the jobs held by 1974 qualifiers who replied to us in 1987 and who had at some time been substantive NHS registrars in general surgery. Of these, 86.2 per cent were engaged in some form of surgical work, including three in general practice combined with a surgical commitment. Fifty (34.5 per cent) were NHS consultants, all but two in surgical disciplines. Seventeen (11.7 per cent) were abroad, of whom fourteen were in surgical work; thirteen (9.0 per cent) were in academic posts, including research assistants and lecturers, and nine (6.2 per cent) were principals in general practice. Forty-four (30.3 per cent) were senior registrars in surgical disciplines and seven (4.8 per cent) were still surgical registrars.

The available information for 1977 qualifiers is less interesting in this respect, as it extends to only nine years after qualifying. At that stage, 7.4 per cent of the 175 respondents who had been substantive registrars in general surgery were abroad, 22.3 per cent were surgical senior registrars (including two senior registrars in dental surgery) and 31.4 per cent were still surgical registrars. Interestingly 17.1 per cent were in academic appointments, all of which were surgical if one post in gastroenterology is included. This is a further indication, as in the case of medicine, that many such posts are transient and are held at an earlier stage than thirteen years after qualifying; but the figures in Tables 11.4 and 11.5 show that nine years after qualifying a higher proportion of 1977 qualifiers held academic surgery posts than did 1974 qualifiers. This tends to support the impression of an expansion in the number of academic and research posts available at the equivalent of registrar or senior registrar level.

12 Individual specialties
Psychiatry

CAREER CHOICES

Table 12.1 shows that at all stages after qualifying, and for both 1974 and 1977 qualifiers, considerably more women than men put psychiatry as their first career choice, and for both men and women there was a steady rise in interest in the specialty during the ten years after leaving medical school.

Among 1974 qualifiers, as shown in Table 3.13 (p. 56), there were fifty-eight first choices, corrected for ties, for psychiatry in 1975, and six years later thirty-nine of these choices persisted, out of a new total of seventy-eight choices. This 67 per cent persistence compares with 81 per cent for general practice choices, 59 per cent for surgical choices, 42 per cent for obstetrics and gynaecology, 40 per cent for medical choices, and 33 per cent for paediatrics.

Table 12.1 Psychiatry: percentages of first choices of career (corrected for ties) at two-yearly intervals after qualifying

Year of qualifying		*Years after qualifying*						
		1	*3*	*5*	*7*	*9*	*11*	*13*
1974	Men	3.4	3.5	3.8	4.1	4.0	4.2	4.1
	Women	3.9	4.6	5.8	6.5	6.9	6.7	6.9
	Total	3.5[a]	3.8	4.3	4.8	4.8	4.9	4.9
1977	Men	2.9	3.3	3.7	3.8	3.9		
	Women	5.3	6.8	7.1	7.9	7.9		
	Total	3.7[a]	4.5	4.8	5.2	5.3		

Note: a Slightly different from originally published figures due to rounding and correction for ties

Of the initial choices for psychiatry which did not persist, eleven transferred to general practice, three to community medicine or community health, and one each to a variety of other interests. The gains to psychiatry during the six years after pre-registration were mainly from general practice (twenty) and medicine (fourteen).

Among individual medical schools, the range in the percentage of first choices for psychiatry at the pre-registration stage, in most of the years that we surveyed, was from 7 or 8 per cent to 1 per cent or nil. The highest percentages were 14.6 per cent from St George's in 1979 and 10.9 per cent from Leicester in 1980.

In five of the eight years St George's was among the top three medical schools for psychiatry career choices; Birmingham and Aberdeen were among the top three on three occasions, and University College Hospital twice. Leicester featured only in the 1980 and 1983 surveys and was among the top three on both occasions. The three medical schools with the lowest percentages of first choices for psychiatry included St Thomas' in four of the eight years, and in two years each St Mary's, Charing Cross Hospital, Aberdeen, the Royal Free, Westminster, Middlesex, and the University of Wales College of Medicine. It will be noted that during the decade a number of medical schools featured as both high and low producers of potential psychiatrists, Aberdeen being three times in the top and twice in the bottom trio.

PSYCHIATRY EXPERIENCE

Table 12.2 shows the number of times that posts of different grades and types, including general practice combined with psychiatry, were held by respondents regardless of whether they initially or subsequently gave psychiatry as a career choice. Multiple posts of the same grade and type, held by the same person, are counted only once in the table. In this respect the table is comparable to those presented for surgery (Tables 11.2 and 11.3).

The 1977 qualifiers had had less time to progress than the 1974 qualifiers, but allowing for this the findings are fairly similar for the two cohorts except that 'other' experience, which includes work abroad, was less common among the later qualifiers. Academic posts were much more often held by men than women. Part-time work featured in almost every type of appointment, part-time registrarships being considerably more frequent among 1977 than 1974 respondents.

Table 12.2 Psychiatry posts held by 1974 and 1977 qualifiers by 1987 and 1986 respectively[a]

Year of qualifying		SHO			Registrar			Senior registrar			Consultant			Academic			GP principal/ Psychiatry	Clinical asst[b]			Other/ unknown[c]		
		FT	*PT*	*Loc*	*FT*	*PT*	*Loc*	*FT*	*PT*	*Loc*	*FT*	*PT*	*Loc*	*FT*	*PT*	*Loc*		*FT*	*PT*	*Loc*	*FT*	*PT*	*Loc*
1974	Men	248	0	9	71	0	6	50	2	7	37	1	7	24	2	0	11	0	1	1	42	1	1
	Women	117	9	4	44	9	5	22	8	5	12	4	3	4	3	1	6	2	17	2	10	12	2
	Total	365	9	13	115	9	11	72	10	12	49	5	10	28	5	1	17	2	18	3	52	13	3
	%[d]	16.1			5.1			3.2			2.2			1.2									
1977	Men	352	0	11	77	3	9	39	3	7	18	0	4	19	1	1	15[e]	0	1	0	27	1	4
	Women	236	9	19	79	16	11	27	7	4	12	0	4	4	0	0	5	1	14	2	10	7	5
	Total	588	9	30	156	19	20	66	10	11	30	0	8	23	1	1	20	1	15	2	37	8	9
	%[d]	19.7			5.2			1.0						0.8									

Notes: a Figures are numbers of posts
b Not including GP principals but including some posts combined with GP locums and/or work in other specialties
c Mainly posts held abroad
d Percentage of number of respondents
e Including two in Canada

Table 12.3 Psychiatry posts held nine years after qualifying (including part-time and locum posts)[a]

Year of qualifying		*SHO*	*Reg.*	*SR*	*Cons.*	*Academic*	*GP/ Psych.*	*Clinical asst.*	*Other/ unknown*	*Total*
1974	Men	1	3	22	18	10	9[b]	0	9	72
	Women	1	7	9	6	1	2[c]	4	6	36
	Total	2	10	31	24	11	11	4	15	108
	%		9	29	22	10	10			
1977	Men	3	6	18	16	12	11[d]	0	11	77
	Women	1	15	20	8	2	3[e]	7	4	60
	Total	4	21	38	24	14	14	7	15	137
	%		15	28	18	10	10			

Notes: a Figures are numbers of posts with percentages of total posts shown
b Including three GP/clinical assistants in mental subnormality and one GP/clinical assistant in forensic psychiatry
c Including one GP/clinical assistant in psychogeriatrics
d Including three GP/clinical assistants in psychogeriatrics, one GP/clinical assistant in mental subnormality, one GP/clinical assistant in psychotherapy and one GP/clinical assistant with an interest in drug abuse
e Including one GP/clinical assistant in mental subnormality and one GP/clinical assistant in psychiatry and psychosexual counselling

Table 12.4 Psychiatry posts held by 1974 qualifiers at latest reply in 1987 (including part-time and locum posts)

	SHO	*Reg.*	*SR*	*Cons.*	*Academic*	*GP/ clinical asst.*	*Clinical asst.*	*Other/ unknown*	*Total*
Psychiatry	2	2	10[a]	23	8	5	3	10	63
Child/adolescent psychiatry	–	–	2	12	1	–	1[c]	1	17
Psychiatry of the elderly	–	–	–	3	–	–	1	–	4
Forensic psychiatry	–	–	1	2	–	1	–	–	4
Mental subnormality	–	–	1	–	–	2	1[d]	–	4
Psychotherapy/psychoanalysis	–	–	–	7	–	2[b]	2[e]	2	13
Total	2	2	14	47	9	10	8	13	105

Notes: a Includes one combined with MRC post
b Includes one combined with psychosexual medicine
c Combined with GP locums
d Combined with family planning
e Both combined with private practice

Table 12.5 Psychiatry posts held abroad (1974 and 1977 qualifiers)

Year of qualifying		*No. of doctors with one or more psychiatry posts abroad*	*EC countries*	*Other Europe*	*Australia*	*New Zealand*	*Canada*	*USA*	*Other*	*Total*	*Academic posts*	*Posts of over 2 yrs*	*Posts of over 3 yrs*
1974	Men	36	4 (2)	1	9 (3)	7 (1)	11 (8)	18 (2)	7 (4)	57	10 (3)	7 (5)	6
	Women	14	3	0	17 (6)	2	4 (2)	1 (1)	0	27	3 (2)	2 (1)	5 (3)
	Total	50	7	1	26	9	15	19	7	84	13	9	11
1977	Men	19	1	1	11 (1)	4	5 (1)	3 (1)	2	27	1 (1)	0	3
	Women	10	4	2	10	2	0	1	2	21	0	0	2
	Total	29	5	3	21	6	5	4	4	48	1	0	5

Note: Numbers in parentheses are posts held by doctors becoming senior registrars and/or consultants in psychiatry in UK

Table 12.6 Progress in relation to career choice: psychiatry

Year of qualifying	*Known to have been non-locum SR or consultant by time of latest reply*				No. (%) choosing psychiatry 1 and/or 3 years after qualifying who had not become a non-locum SR and/or consultant in psychiatry
	Known first career choices for psychiatry (tied or untied) 1 and/or 3 years after qualifying	*Not choosing psychiatry 1 or 3 years after qualifying*	*Missing replies and/or choices not given*	*Total no. (%) of respondents*	
1974	49	7	22	78[a] (3.4)	55 (53)
1977	62	10	1	73[b] (2.4)	101 (62)

Notes: a By 1987
b By 1986

CAREER PROGRESS

Table 12.3 compares the qualifiers of 1974 and 1977 who held psychiatry posts in April 1983 and April 1986 respectively. At this stage the proportions of post-holders in the senior registrar grade were the same, but a higher percentage of the 1977 qualifiers than those of 1974 were in the registrar grade and a lower percentage had become consultants. The percentages in academic posts, and in general practice, were the same for the two cohorts.

Table 12.4 shows the posts held by those 1974 qualifiers who replied to us in 1987 and who were working in psychiatry at that time. Of those known to be working in the specialty, 45 per cent were consultants thirteen years after qualifying; of these forty-seven people twenty-three were consultants in general psychiatry, twelve in child and adolescent psychiatry, three in psychiatry of the elderly, two in forensic psychiatry, seven in psychotherapy/psychoanalysis and none in mental subnormality.

Table 12.5 shows psychiatry experience abroad: 2.2 per cent of 1974 qualifiers and only 1.0 per cent of 1977 qualifiers were known to have held such posts, and the most striking difference was in the reduced uptake of posts in Canada and the USA. Academic posts abroad in psychiatry were more often held by men than women. Of the fourteen academic posts shown, seven were in the USA, five in Canada, one in Australia and one in the EC. The numbers in parentheses in the table are posts held by doctors who subsequently became senior registrars and/or consultants in the UK.

Of the seventy-nine doctors shown, fifty-one had held one psychiatry post abroad, sixteen had held two, and twelve had held more than two, including three doctors with five and one doctor with eight posts abroad.

SENIOR REGISTRARS AND CONSULTANTS IN PSYCHIATRY

Table 12.6 shows that 63 per cent of 1974 qualifiers who became senior registrars and/or consultants in psychiatry, and 85 per cent of 1977 qualifiers who did so, had given psychiatry as their first choice of career one and/or three years after qualifying. This apparent difference is at least partly explained by the fact that among 1974 qualifiers there were twenty-two who either did not reply to us one or three years after qualifying, or did not give a clear career choice in those years, whereas information about early career choices was available for all but one of the 1977 respondents.

Nine years after qualifying, 62 per cent of the 1977 qualifiers who gave psychiatry as their first career choice at the pre-registration stage were not known to have become senior registrars and/or consultants; after thirteen years, 53 per cent of the comparable respondents who qualified in 1974 were not known to have had substantive posts in these grades. The time taken to become a substantive senior registrar in psychiatry, by the forty-six male 1974 qualifiers for whom dates are available, ranged from four to eleven years (mean 6.4 years). For twenty-five women the range was four to thirteen years (mean 7.4 years).

Among 1977 qualifiers, the time taken by thirty-nine men who gave dates ranged from four to nine years (nine years being the time of the latest questionnaire: mean 5.7 years); for the thirty-three women the range was also four to nine years (mean 6.6 years).

In both years men became senior registrars more rapidly than women, which is in contrast to the situation shown in anaesthetics from our data (Chapter 13). Once again, the 1977 figures are constrained by the limit to our follow-up, so that earlier achievers predominate. For all hospital specialties combined, the mean time taken by 1974 respondents to achieve senior registrar status was 7.4 years for men and 7.3 years for women; for 1977 respondents it was 6.6 years for men and 6.2 years for women.

The time taken to achieve consultant status in psychiatry, by thirty-eight male 1974 qualifiers, ranged from seven to thirteen years (mean 9.6 years); for the fifteen women the range was also seven to thirteen years (mean 9.7 years). For seventeen male 1977 qualifiers who gave dates of appointment, the range was seven to nine years (mean 8.1 years); for the twelve women the range was seven to ten years (mean 8.8 years). These figures compare with a mean time to achieve consultant status in all hospital specialties combined among our 1974 qualifiers of 10.1 years for both men and women, and among 1977 qualifiers of 8.3 years for men and 8.1 years for women.

Table 12.7 shows the numbers of posts of various types, other than psychiatry, held by respondents who became senior registrars and/or consultants in psychiatry. Most of this experience was of a kind likely to be associated with general practice vocational training, either organized and not completed or self-constructed; that, is general practice, obstetrics and gynaecology, paediatrics, accident and emergency, and medicine.

Table 12.7 Non-psychiatry experience of senior registrars and/or consultants (number of posts)

	1974 qualifiers						*1977 qualifiers*					
	UK posts		*UK locums*		*abroad*		*UK posts*		*UK locums*		*abroad*	
Specialty	*M*	*F*	*M*	*F*	*M*	*F*	*M*	*F*	*M*	*F*	*M*	*F*
Medicine and medical specialties	15	3	2	–	–	1	9	12	2	1	–	–
Neurology	2	–	–	–	–	–	1	2	–	–	–	–
Geriatrics	3	1	1	–	–	–	2	3	–	1	–	–
Paediatrics	7	4	–	1	–	1	5	6	–	1	–	–
Obstetrics & gynaecology	4	5	–	–	–	–	6	8	–	–	–	–
Surgery and surgical specialties	2	1	–	–	1	–	5	1	–	–	–	–
Accident & emergency	4	2	–	1	–	–	5	7	–	–	1	–
Anaesthetics	1	–	–	–	–	–	1	1	–	1	–	–
Radiotherapy	1	1	–	–	–	–	–	–	–	–	–	–
Pathology	1	–	–	–	–	1	–	–	–	–	–	–
General practice	5	9	–	2	2	1	3	9	–	1	1	–
Community medicine/health	–	5	–	–	–	–	3	1	–	–	–	–
Third World medicine	–	–	–	–	2	–	–	–	–	–	1	1
Other/not known	1	2	–	–	–	2	1	1	–	–	1	1
Total	46	33	3	4	5	6	41	51	2	5	4	2

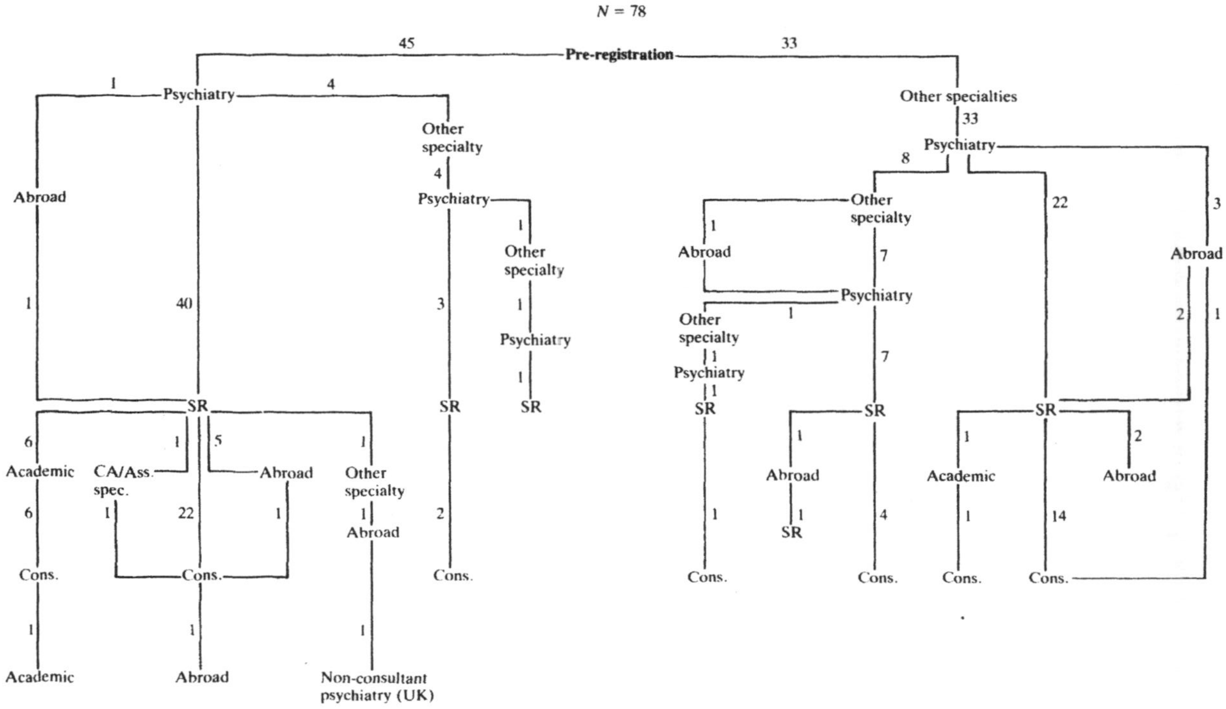

Figure 12.1 Career paths of 1974 qualifiers becoming senior registrars and/or consultants in psychiatry
Note: **The numbers of senior registrars shown include four doctors with academic posts only at senior registrar level**

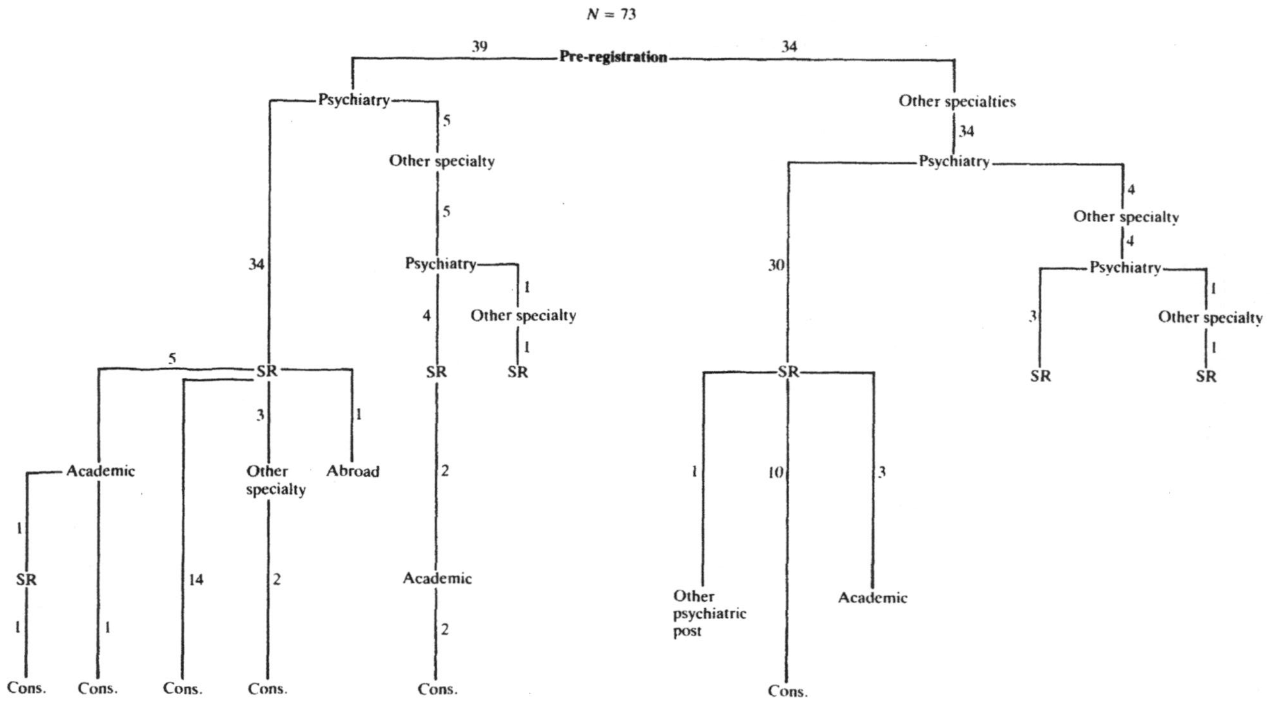

Figure 12.2 Career paths of 1977 qualifiers becoming senior registrars and/or consultants in psychiatry

Note: **The numbers of senior registrars shown include one doctor with academic post only at senior registrar level**

A few respondents had considerably greater medical experience, for example two with MD, MRCP, and four respondents had worked in the Third World. 'Other' experience included the Armed Forces. To our knowledge 53 per cent of 1974 qualifiers and 47 per cent of 1977 qualifiers had not obtained any post-graduate experience beyond the pre-registration year except in psychiatry, before becoming senior registrars and/or consultants in psychiatry.

A somewhat simplified representation of the routes by which respondents reached senior registrar and consultant posts is given in Figures 12.1 and 12.2. It will be seen from Table 12.5 (numbers in parentheses) that considerably fewer psychiatry posts abroad were held by 1977 qualifiers than by 1974 qualifiers en route to a senior registrar or consultant post. In fact, among those who had held senior registrar and/or consultant posts there were eleven men and six women from the 1974 cohort who gained psychiatry experience abroad, and only three men from the 1977 cohort.

Nine years after qualifying 53 per cent of the 1977 group who pursued psychiatry alone after the pre-registration year had become consultants, compared to 31 per cent of those with experience outside the specialty. Thirteen years after qualifying the proportions becoming consultants among the 1974 group were 62 and 73 per cent for those with and those without extraneous experience.

Of those respondents with senior registrar posts in psychiatry, 42 per cent of 1974 qualifiers and 37 per cent of 1977 qualifiers held these posts in the region of their medical school; 36 per cent and 40 per cent respectively held their psychiatry consultant posts in the region of their medical school. From the two cohorts, 53 per cent and 60 per cent of respondents respectively were known to have held senior registrar and consultant posts in psychiatry in the same region, and for 30 per cent and 27 per cent respectively this was the region of their medical school. Among the 1974 respondents higher proportions of men than women had held senior registrar and/or consultant posts in psychiatry in their medical school regions, but the reverse was true among the 1977 respondents in psychiatry, and for all hospital specialties combined. Taking the sexes and cohorts together, the figures for psychiatry in this paragraph are very similar to those for all hospital specialties combined (Chapter 6).

Among the 1974 qualifiers from Scottish medical schools 58 per cent of those with senior registrar posts in psychiatry and 63 per cent of those with consultant posts in psychiatry held the post concerned in England and Wales. Among the Scottish 1977 qualifiers 35 per cent of psychiatry senior registrar posts and 44 per cent of psychiatry consultant posts were in England and Wales. From medical schools in England and Wales three senior registrar posts in psychiatry (5 per cent) and one consultant post (3 per cent) were held in Scotland by 1974 qualifiers and none in either grade was held by 1977 qualifiers.

PART-TIME EMPLOYMENT

Among those who had been senior registrars and/or consultants, from both cohorts, twenty-four women and six men were known to have held one or more part-time appointments of some kind, at some stage. Ten of these women had been full-time senior registrars before recording any part-time work; nine of them were working part-time when they last replied to us and one, who had also been working part-time, had recently died. One was a part-time consultant and one a part-time senior lecturer; four were part-time senior registrars, one of whom also held an academic post; two were clinical assistants, one following a move with her husband and one in psycho-geriatrics following work abroad; one was working part-time in psychiatry in Australia. The latest replies from the other fourteen women indicated that two were full-time consultants, both having been full-time registrars and senior registrars with previous part-time clinical assistantships; two were part-time consultants, one in psychotherapy, in both cases following part-time senior registrarships interrupted for maternity; two, of whom one was in mental subnormality, were full-time senior registrars following various part-time appointments including SHO, registrar, clinical assistant and general practitioner; eight were part-time senior registrars, three in child psychiatry, in three of the eight cases after full-time registrarships and in five cases following part-time registrar and other experience including the Women Doctors' Retainer Scheme, clinical assistantship and a variety of work outside psychiatry.

Of the six men with known part-time work, three had held part-time academic posts in the course of training, one had been a part-time registrar between full-time posts, one had been part-time senior registrar and one, in psychotherapy, held his first part-time post as a consultant. Three of the six were full-time consultants when last replying to us, one was a full-time senior registrar and one held an administrative post related to psychiatry.

COMMENT

Much of the literature on staffing and training in psychiatry has concentrated on recruitment problems, for example Francis Creed's 1979 symposium 'Who puts medical students off psychiatry?' (Angold 1979), the Cambridge Conference of 1982 (Walton 1986) and John Birtchnell's recent study (1987) for the Society of Clinical Psychiatrists. Peter Brook (1976) did much work on 'Where do psychiatrists come from?', looking at the output of psychiatrists from British medical schools from 1961 to 1970. He concluded that discrepancies were very great and that no ready explanations for these were forthcoming. Our findings would support this, although it must seem that the combination of an active clinical service and a strong academic unit with a concern for the organization of good training in the region is, as with other specialties, a powerful influence.

The staffing implications of our data are less clear than in some specialties because of the development of special interests and sub-specialization within psychiatry. This, and the changing social climate, uncovers needs that have apparently not been fully met, so that the 'ideal' numbers of consultants to serve a given population in, for example, forensic psychiatry, psychiatry of the elderly, child and adolescent psychiatry and drug and alcohol dependence are open to revision. It would be unwise to seek too much detailed enlightenment from the fairly small numbers in this study. For instance, it happened that seven of our 1974 qualifiers had become consultants in psychotherapy and none in mental subnormality; the England and Wales figures for the three years 1983/84 to 1985/86 inclusive show that thirty-five paid consultants were newly appointed in mental subnormality and seventeen in psychotherapy. Psychiatry of the elderly is not shown separately in the Department of Health tables, although it was surveyed by Wattis *et al.* (1981). The number of paid consultants appointed in mental illness including psychogeriatrics, over the three years was 198, in child and adolescent psychiatry 73 and in forensic psychiatry 20. This average annual rate of about 115 consultant appointments is augmented by the numbers appointed in Scotland and Northern Ireland, and the appointments to academic posts with consultant status. There are also opportunities in private practice and abroad, although the export of graduates should be balanced by the appointment of some overseas doctors to career posts in the UK. The experience of overseas qualified doctors with and after the MRC Psych was reviewed by Bhate *et al.* (1986).

Audrey Ward's (1984) study of psychiatrists who passed the

MRC Psych in 1975-7 showed a similar level of involvement in the specialty to our findings, with women progressing more slowly than men and frequently working part-time. The reduced uptake of posts abroad among our 1977 qualifiers compared to those of 1974 was not confined to psychiatry (Chapter 7). It almost certainly indicates reduced opportunity and reluctance to depart from an increasingly prescriptive pattern of training. Altogether, and if recent consultant expansion is sustained, the prospective *total* number of career opportunities in the psychiatry specialties would accommodate approximately 4 per cent of qualifiers from UK medical schools, although NHS career outlets in psychiatry appear to represent almost 6 per cent of all career outlets in the NHS.

Experience of psychiatry among doctors qualifying in 1974 and 1977 was considerable, and although these years are likely to be fairly typical, the amount of contact with the specialty among young doctors has very probably increased with the development and popularity of vocational training for general practice. Much of the non-psychiatry experience described here, and many of the SHO posts shown in Table 12.2, were part of a tentative or uncompleted general practice training. This opportunity to find out about psychiatry at first hand may lead to some recruitment into the specialty, but perhaps even more likely to do so is a period of time spent in general practice, which brings realization to how many patients require more than help with merely physical problems.

When settled on a career in psychiatry, progress appears from our data to be marginally more rapid than is the average for hospital specialties in general. It was slower for 1977 qualifiers than for those who qualified in 1974, as judged after nine years from leaving medical school. Also, women progressed more slowly than men on average, but this may be attributable at least partly to the fact that part-time training is relatively common in psychiatry. In England and Wales at 30 September 1986, 5.9 per cent of registrars in the psychiatry specialties and 12.1 per cent of senior registrars were part-time compared to 2.9 per cent of registrars and 7.7 per cent of senior registrars in all hospital specialties combined. The next highest proportions of part-time staff after psychiatry were in anaesthetics and pathology, with 5.9 per cent and 5.4 per cent part-time registrars and 8.0 per cent and 9.3 per cent part-time senior registrars respectively. The experiences of the respondents reported in this study confirm the general impression that psychiatry as a specialty tends to be considerate to the needs of doctors with domestic responsibilities. Movement between regions during training was common in this survey, as for other hospital specialties. Fewer of the 1977 respondents than those of 1974 migrated from Scottish medical schools to England and Wales for senior registrar and consultant posts.

13 Individual specialties

Anaesthetics

CAREER CHOICE

Career choices for anaesthetics are given in Chapter 3, and these include choices for anaesthetics combined with intensive care or pain therapy, and the very occasional preferences for intensive care or pain therapy alone. General practice combined with anaesthetics is not included as a career choice in these figures.

Over the whole decade of our surveys the lowest percentage of first choices for anaesthetics at the pre-registration stage was 3.8 per cent among 1975 qualifiers, and the highest was 6.0 per cent among 1976 and 1980 qualifiers (Chapter 3). The mean for eight years was 5.3 per cent. For both 1974 and 1977 qualifiers, there was a gain in the number of potential recruits to the specialty during the first few years after qualifying, with a tendency for the number of preferences to level off thereafter.

Among 1974 qualifiers (Table 3.13), the actual number of first choices for anaesthetics, corrected for ties, was 70 at the pre-registration stage. Six years later, in 1981, there were 103 such choices. Of these 103 choices, 45 were from among the original 70, that is 64 per cent of the first choices for anaesthetics had persisted for six years. This was a lower persistence rate than for general practice, and slightly lower than for psychiatry, but substantially higher than for other specialties. During these seven years after qualifying twenty first choices of career had changed *to* anaesthetics from surgery, eighteen from general practice, ten from medicine, and nine from other specialty choices. There were sixteen changes of first choice *from* anaesthetics to general practice, two to medicine, and eight to other career choices (all figures rounded to the nearest whole number).

Although there were considerable variations between medical schools in the numbers of graduates giving anaesthetics as first choice of career, there was little evidence of consistency. For 1974 qualifiers the medical schools showing the highest number of choices for anaesthetics were Bristol, King's College Hospital and Westminster Hospital; the lowest were Charing Cross Hospital and University College Hospital. For 1977 qualifiers the highest ranking schools were Aberdeen, Edinburgh and Leeds; the lowest were St George's Hospital and Middlesex Hospital. For the eight years that we surveyed, there were two medical schools which featured three times among the three highest-ranking in terms of career preferences for anaesthetics, but one of these also featured on one occasion among the three lowest-ranking. Conversely two medical schools featured three times among the three lowest-ranking for anaesthetics preferences, and one of these also featured in one year among the three highest-ranking.

ANAESTHETICS EXPERIENCE

Table 13.1 shows varieties of anaesthetics experience obtained by 1974 and 1977 qualifiers, including locum posts, GP/anaesthetics appointments, and posts abroad or in HM Forces. As with comparable tables in previous chapters, this table shows numbers of holders of posts of various types, rather than the total number of posts held: that is a doctor who held more than one full-time SHO post would be counted once in the full-time SHO column, and would be counted again, once, in the full-time register column if he or she had held one or more full-time registrar posts, and so on.

Up to the times of our latest surveys, 12.3 per cent of 1974 qualifiers were known to have had anaesthetics experience of some kind, and 12.5 per cent of 1977 qualifiers had done so. There is an obvious difference between the two cohorts in the number of consultant posts obtained, but otherwise, for men and women combined, the percentages in various grades and types of appointment are very similar except for a lower percentage of 1977 qualifiers having held 'other' posts which consist mainly of anaesthetics appointments abroad. Also notable is the difference between the numbers of men and women anaesthetists in academic appointments, among both 1974 and 1977 respondents.

Table 13.2 shows anaesthetics posts held outside the UK by male and female 1974 qualifiers. The table counts the total number of posts held abroad; some doctors had held more than one post abroad, and had been to more than one part of the world. Table 13.3 shows how many male and female doctors had held different numbers of posts outside the UK.

Table 13.1 Anaesthetics posts held by 1974 and 1977 qualifiers by 1987 and 1986 respectively, with totals and percentages of respondents

Year of qualifying		*SHO*			*Registrar*			*Senior registrar*			*Consultant*			*Academic*			*Clinical asst.*			*Other*[a]		
		FT	*PT*	*Loc*	*FT*	*PT*	*Loc*	*FT*	*PT*	*Loc*	*FT*	*PT*	*Loc*	*FT*	*PT*	*Loc*	*FT*	*PT*	*Loc*	*FT*	*PT*	*Loc*
1974	Men	176	0	4	120	0	18	76	0	19	57	0	9	27	0	2	1	5	1	78	1	9
	Women	57	1	1	29	3	7	12	4	5	9	2	6	2	0	0	0	11	2	15	2	3
	Total	233	1	5	149	3	25	88	4	24	66	2	15	29	0	2	1	16	3	93	3	12
	%	10.3			6.6			3.9			2.9			1.3						4.1		
1977	Men	218	0	12	134	0	25	93	0	18	39	0	10	27[b]	0	0	0	5	3	63	1	9
	Women	117	1	8	67	4	14	25	2	8	7	0	7	4	2	0	0	11	3	19	5	2
	Total	335	1	20	201	4	39	118	2	26	46	0	17	31	2	0	0	16	6	82	6	11
	%	11.2			6.7			3.9			1.5			1.0						2.7		

Notes: a Mainly posts held abroad

b Including two honorary senior registrars

Also: Six post-registration house officers, four research registrars, one research senior registrar, one locum associate specialist, one part-time CMO, two GP anaesthetists and one part-time hospital practitioner

Source: Parkhouse and Ellin 1990b

Table 13.2 Anaesthetics posts held abroad (1974 and 1977 qualifiers)

Year of qualifying		*EC countries*	*Other Europe*	*Australia*	*New Zealand*	*Canada*	*USA*	*Other*	*Total*
1974	Men	21	11	15	10	31	23	21	132
	Women	4	0	0	1	5	1	19	30
	Total	25	11	15	11	36	24	40	162
1977	Men	11	4	16	24	19	17	23	114
	Women	3	2	6	4	7	1	8	31
	Total	14	6	22	28	26	18	31	145

Source: Parkhouse and Ellin 1990b

Table 13.3 Numbers of anaesthetics posts abroad, held by 1974 and 1977 qualifiers (with cumulative frequency)

Year of qualifying		*Number of overseas posts*								
		1	*2*	*3*	*4*	*5*	*6*	*7*	*total*	*Cumulative frequency*
1974	Men	53	14	9	2	2	1	0	81	132
	Women	10	6	1	0	1	0	0	18	30
	Total	63	20	10	2	3	1	0	99[a]	162
1977	Men	57	11	4	4	0	0	1	77	114
	Women	13	4	2	1	0	0	0	20	31
	Total	70	15	6	5	0	0	1	97[b]	145

Notes: a 4.4% of 2,272 respondents
b 3.2% of 2,988 respondents
Source: Parkhouse and Ellin 1990b

Altogether 4.4 per cent of 1974 qualifiers and 3.2 per cent of 1977 qualifiers were known to have held one or more anaesthetics posts abroad. There is an appreciable sex difference: among 1974 qualifiers 4.9 per cent of men and 2.9 per cent of women were known to have held such posts, and among 1977 qualifiers, 3.8 per cent of men and 2.0 per cent of women.

Most doctors had held one or two posts abroad, but a few had held as many as six or seven. Most of the posts were of fairly short duration; posts were held abroad for two years or more by twenty-seven 1974 qualifiers and eleven 1977 qualifiers.

The most popular individual countries for anaesthetics posts among 1974 qualifiers were Canada, the USA and Australia, and for 1977 qualifiers, New Zealand, Canada and Australia. Although the numbers are fairly small, the women doctors in both cohorts were more likely than the men to have worked elsewhere in the world than the highly developed and traditionally popular countries specifically noted in Table 13.2. For 1974 qualifiers, sixteen anaesthetics posts abroad were classed as academic appointments, eleven in the USA, three in Canada, one in New Zealand and one elsewhere. For the 1977 qualifiers, fourteen anaesthetics posts abroad were classed as academic, eight in the USA, four in Canada and two elsewhere. All but two of these twenty-nine posts were held by men.

It must again be remembered that the 1977 qualifiers had not been followed for as long as those of 1974, but considering the fact that the earlier cohort was smaller, these figures, together with the numbers of 'other' posts shown in Table 13.1, suggest a reduced uptake of posts abroad, including academic appointments, among the later qualifiers.

Table 13.4 shows that, comparing doctors known to have become senior registrars and/or consultants in anaesthetics with others in anaesthetics who had worked abroad, the former were more likely to have taken academic appointments overseas, to have travelled less frequently and for shorter periods, and less often to the more undeveloped parts of the world. This might indicate a number of things: for instance, that a sense of freedom to roam and explore is likely to go with an open-minded view of the future, rather than a set design to achieve consultant status in the UK, or that the probability of achieving this status, through a senior registrarship, is diminished by 'stepping off the ladder'. The increased popularity of posts in New Zealand and Australia among 1977 qualifiers which shows in Table 13.2 is seen from Table 13.4 to be largely among doctors who subsequently became senior registrars and/or consultants.

Table 13.4 Anaesthetics experience abroad of respondents known and not known to have become senior registrars and/or consultants in anaesthetics

	Year of qualifying	*Europe*	*Australia and New Zealand*	*USA and Canada*	*Other countries*	*Total*	*More than one post abroad*	*Academic posts abroad*	*Posts abroad for 2 years or more*
Doctors known to have become SR or consultant in anaesthetics	1974	21	3	25	13	62	11	10	6
	1977	7	22	27	10	66	8	12	0
	Total	28	25	52	23	128	19	22	6
Doctors not known to have become SR or consultant in anaesthetics	1974	15	23	35	27	100	25	6	21
	1977	13	28	17	21	79	19	2	11
	Total	28	51	52	48	179	44	8	32
	Total	56	76	104	71	307	63	30	38

Source: Parkhouse and Ellin 1990b

Table 13.5 Anaesthetics posts held nine years after qualifying (including part-time and locum posts)

Year of qualifying		*SHO*	*Reg.*	*SR*	*Cons.*	*Academic*	*GP/ anaes.*	*Other/ unknown*	*Total*
1974[a]	Men	3	7	47	14	8	6[c]	14	99
	Women	0	5	9	4	1	2	5	26
	Total	3	12	56	18	9	8	19	125
1977[b]	Men	0	11	48	27	12	11[e]	17	126
	Women	2	6	19	7	2	1	14[f]	51
	Total	2	17	67	34	14	12	31	177

Notes: a Based on replies from 1,514 men and 573 women
b Based on replies from 1,680 men and 869 women
c Including one in Canada and one in Channel Islands
d Including one part-time clinical assistant
e Including one with sessions in obstetrics and gynaecology; one with work in acupuncture and one GP with dental anaesthesia
f Including six part-time clinical assistants, one with sessions in blood transfusion

Source: Parkhouse and Ellin 1990b

Table 13.6 Anaesthetics posts held by 1974 qualifiers at latest information in 1987 (including part-time and locum posts)

	SHO	*Registrar*	*SR*	*Consultant*	*Academic*	*GP/ anaesthetics*	*Other/ unknown*	*Total*
Men	1[a]	1[b]	5	57	9	7[c]	9	89
Women	0	0	3	13	0	2	6[d]	24
Total	1	1	8	70	9	9	15	113

Notes: a Latest reply indicates SHO in 1985
b Locum registrar in 1987
c Includes one in Canada, one in Channel Islands and one in Royal Navy
d Includes three part-time clinical assistants
Source: Parkhouse and Ellin 1990b

CAREER PROGRESS

Table 13.5 shows anaesthetics posts held by 1974 and 1977 qualifiers nine years after leaving medical school. It appears that the 1977 qualifiers had made somewhat more rapid progress at this stage, 19 per cent of those with anaesthetics appointments being consultants and 38 per cent being senior registrars, compared to 14 per cent and 45 per cent respectively of the 1974 qualifiers. The difference was mainly among men (21 per cent as consultants, compared to 14 per cent) but altogether these figures have to be seen in a context of rapid change: for example if the 1986 situation of 1977 qualifiers is assessed on all the questionnaire returns, some of which arrived in late 1986 or early 1987, rather than on the jobs held specifically in April 1986, the proportion of anaesthetic post-holders who were consultants already rises to 27 per cent.

Table 13.6 shows types of posts held by 1974 qualifiers who replied to us in 1987, and whose latest reported post was in anaesthetics. The disparity in the number of male and female occupants of academic posts is again evident. It is also interesting that there is a wide spread of posts, from SHO level to consultant level, even eleven to thirteen years after qualifying. This reflects partly the broad range of other experience obtained by some doctors before settling to a career in anaesthetics, and partly the difficulty with examinations and promotion which some doctors encounter.

SENIOR REGISTRARS AND CONSULTANTS IN ANAESTHETICS

For 1974 qualifiers who gave the dates of their first substantive appointments, the time taken to become a senior registrar in anaesthetics ranged from five to twelve years (mean 6.9 years). The time taken to become a consultant ranged from seven to thirteen years (mean 9.8 years). The mean time taken by seventy-two men who gave valid dates to reach senior registrarship was 6.9 years; for the sixteen women it was 6.6 years. These figures compare with mean times taken by 1974 respondents, in all hospital specialties combined, of 7.4 years for men and 7.3 years for women to achieve substantive senior registrar status, and 10.1 years for both men and women to achieve substantive consultant status.

For 1977 qualifiers who gave dates of their appointments, the time taken to become a senior registrar in anaesthetics ranged

Table 13.7 Progress in relation to career choice: anaesthetics

	Known to have been non-locum SR or consultant by time of latest reply				
Year of qualifying	*Known first career choices for anaesthetics (tied or untied) 1 and/or 3 years after qualifying*	*Not choosing anaesthetics 1 or 3 years after qualifying*	*Missing replies and/or choices not given*	*Total no. (%) of respondents*	*No. (%) choosing anaesthetics 1 and/or 3 years after qualifying who had not become a non-locum SR and/or consultant in anaesthetics*
1974	68	9	16	93[a] (4.1)	75[b] (52)
1977	101	6	12	119[b] (4.0)	154[b] (60)

Notes: a By 1987
b By 1986
Source: Parkhouse and Ellin 1990b

from four to nine years (mean 6.5 years); the time taken to become a consultant ranged from six to ten years (mean 8.5 years). The mean time taken by ninety-two men to reach senior registrarship was 6.5 years and for twenty-five women it was 6.4 years. For 1977 respondents in all hospital specialties combined, the mean time taken to achieve substantive senior registrar status was 6.6 years for men and 6.2 years for women, and to achieve substantive consultant status 8.3 years for men and 8.1 years for women.

Among the 1974 respondents, progress in anaesthetics seemed to be rather more rapid than that in the hospital specialties generally. The upper limits on all these ranges are determined by the length of time for which qualifiers have been followed; for example, the mean time taken by those 1977 qualifiers who had become consultants within nine years of qualifying is heavily influenced by those who had made rapid progress.

All the above figures exclude holders of academic posts with honorary NHS senior registrar or consultant grading.

Table 13.7 shows that about 4 per cent of the respondents in each cohort had been senior registrars or consultants in anaesthetics by the time of their latest reply. Of these, 73 per cent from the 1974 cohort and 85 per cent from the 1977 cohort had given anaesthetics as a first choice of career one and/or three years after qualifying.

In the 1974 cohort 107 men and 36 women were known to have given anaesthetics as their first choice of career one and/or three years after qualifying. Of these doctors, 54 men (50 per cent) and 14 women (39 per cent) were known to have achieved non-locum senior registrar or consultant status by 1987. For 1977 qualifiers in 1986, the comparable figures were 79 of 164 men (48 per cent) and 22 of 91 women (24 per cent).

Of the 1974 qualifiers who had become senior registrars and/or consultants in anaesthetics in the UK, 27 men (35 per cent) and 5 women (31 per cent) had not to the best of our knowledge had any postgraduate experience beyond the pre-registration year except in anaesthetics — altogether, 32 of 93 doctors (34 per cent). For the 1977 qualifiers, the comparable figure was 54 of 119 doctors (45 per cent) — 42 men (45 per cent) and 12 women (48 per cent).

Table 13.8 shows the numbers and types of posts held by those doctors becoming senior registrars and/or consultants in anaesthetics who did record experience outside the specialty. Substantive appointments in the NHS were most often in accident and emergency, medicine (especially chest medicine and cardiology), obstetrics and gynaecology, paediatrics and general

Table 13.8 Non-anaesthetics experience of senior registrars and/or consultants (number of posts)

	1974 qualifiers						1977 qualifiers					
	UK posts		*UK locums*		*abroad*		*UK posts*		*UK locums*		*abroad*	
Specialty	*M*	*F*	*M*	*F*	*M*	*F*	*M*	*F*	*M*	*F*	*M*	*F*
Medicine and medical specialties	18	4	6	1	1	0	29	9	3	0	0	1
Paediatrics	8	1	2	0	2	0	6	0	1	0	0	0
Accident & emergency	16	3	4	0	2	0	24	7	1	1	0	0
Surgery and surgical specialties	5	1	2	0	3	0	8	3	3	0	2	2
Obstetrics & gynaecology	14	6	1	0	2	0	9	1	1	0	0	0
General practice	2	0	4	0	9	0	8	0	0	0	0	0
Other	8	0	2	2	2	0	9	0	0	1	2	0
Total	71	15	21	3	21	0	93	20	9	2	4	3

Source: Parkhouse and Ellin 1990b

Table 13.9 Non-anaesthetics postgraduate qualifications held by respondents becoming senior registrars and/or consultants in anaesthetics

Year of qualifying		*MRCP pt 1*	*MRCP pt 2*	*FRCS prim.*	*MRCOG pt 1*	*DCH*	*DRCOG*	*MD*	*PhD*	*ECFMG*	*FLEX*	*Other including abroad*
1974	Men	6	2	0	0	2	6	1	1	2	1	4
	Women	1	1	1	0	0	3	0	0	0	0	1
1977	Men	8	7	0	1	1	3	3	2	3	0	0
	Women	1	1	0	0	0	0	0	0	0	0	0

Source: Parkhouse and Ellin 1990b

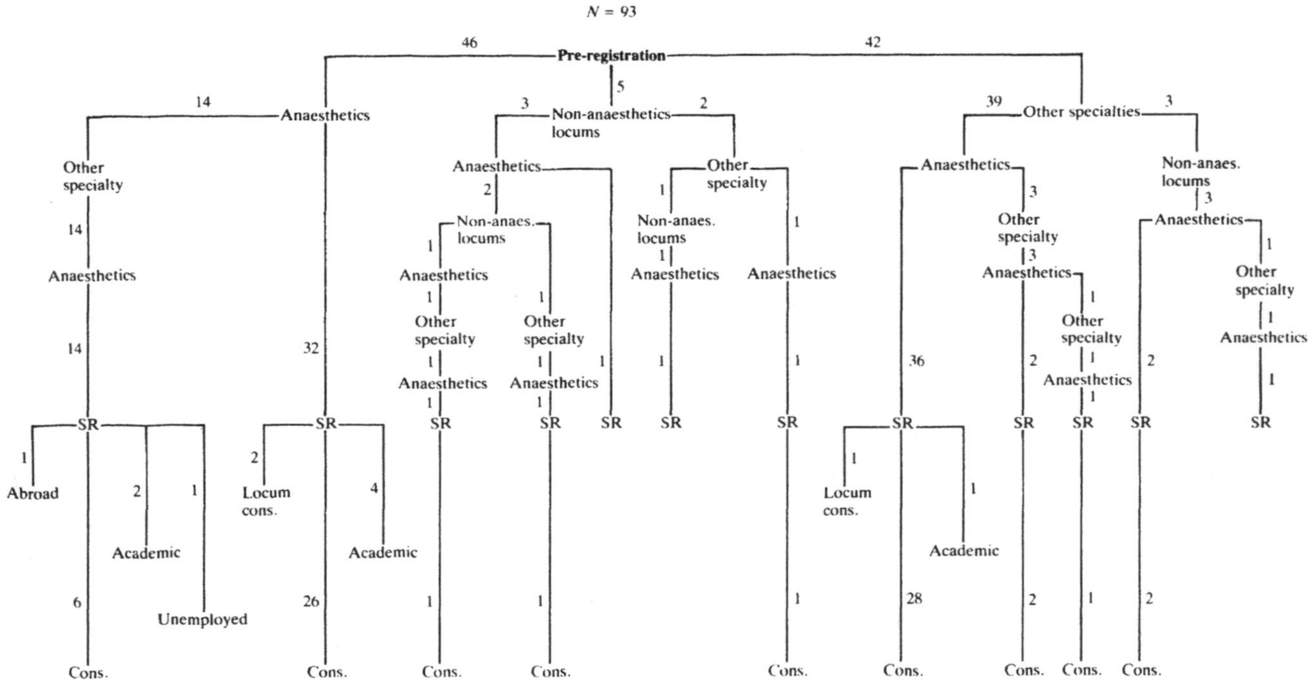

Figure 13.1 Career paths of 1974 qualifiers becoming senior registrars and/or consultants in anaesthetics

Note: The numbers of senior registrars shown include two doctors whose only post at this level was a lectureship with honorary senior registrar status

Source: Parkhouse and Ellin 1990b

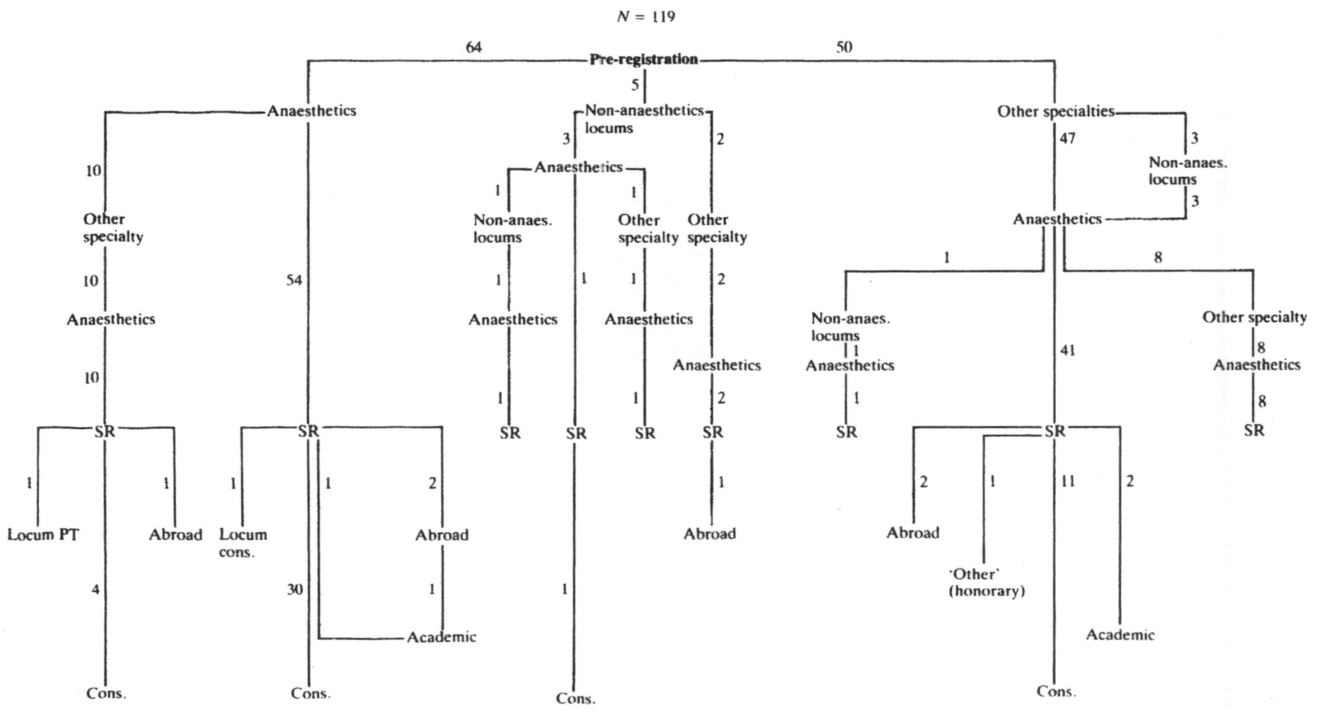

Figure 13.2 Career paths of 1977 qualifiers becoming senior registrars and/or consultants in anaesthetics

Note: **The numbers of senior registrars shown include two doctors whose only post at this level was a lectureship with honorary senior registrar status**

Source: Parkhouse and Ellin 1990b

practice. In a few cases this was noted to be part of a vocational training scheme which was not completed. Some filling-in between regular jobs with locum appointments is apparent, and sometimes experience was obtained abroad either between anaesthetics posts or before settling in the specialty. Taking account of duration as well as number of posts, the most substantial volume of experience outside anaesthetics tended to be medicine; this was more so among 1977 qualifiers than those of 1974, despite a greater concentration on anaesthetics overall in the later cohort.

All but two of the non-anaesthetics posts recorded by all 1974 respondents had been held within nine years of qualifying, indicating that the figures can properly be compared with those for the 1977 respondents. Table 13.9 shows the non-anaesthetics qualifications gained by those who had become senior registrars and/or consultants in anaesthetics; although the numbers are small, they tend to bear out the emphasis on medicine among 1977 qualifiers, especially men.

Figures 13.1 and 13.2 give a general picture of the routes taken towards a senior registrarship in anaesthetics, and the subsequent posts held by those no longer in that grade. The main aim of these diagrams is to separate anaesthetics from non-anaesthetics experience, to show the stages at which non-anaesthetics posts were held, and to give an indication of the uptake of locum appointments outside the specialty, for various reasons, between substantive posts. For simplicity, therefore, all anaesthetics appointments, including part-time posts, locums and posts overseas or in HM Forces, are grouped together.

Among the doctors who had become senior registrars or consultants in anaesthetics, including those who had held locum posts in these grades, there were seven women and five men among the 1974 qualifiers who had at some stage held part-time anaesthetics posts, and six women and two men among the 1977 qualifiers. These individual cases show a wide variety of patterns of experience. Among the women doctors, two were part-time consultants, one having previously been a part-time senior registrar and the other having previously worked abroad; five were part-time senior registrars, two having previously been part-time registrars, three having had breaks in employment for maternity, and two having previously held a variety of part-time locum consultant and other posts; two were part-time clinical assistants; one was a part-time specialist abroad; two had held a succession of part-time locum consultant and other posts before stopping work for family reasons, and one was a part-time 'locum' following a senior registrarship and a break for maternity. Of the male doctors, six had held part-time locum appointments, as consultant, registrar or clinical assistant, for periods of one to nine months and in one case having held fourteen such locum posts, either part-time or full-time at various stages; one male doctor had held a part-time clinical assistantship concurrently with a basic science research appointment.

LOCATION OF SENIOR REGISTRAR AND CONSULTANT POSTS IN ANAESTHETICS

Table 13.10 displays this information for those 1974 and 1977 qualifiers who had obtained substantive senior registrar posts and, in some cases, consultant posts in anaesthetics. Locations of the first substantive posts in these grades are shown in relation to the region of the medical school, and for qualifiers from the London medical schools a post in central London or any of the four Thames regions is regarded as a post in the same region as the medical school.

For 1974 qualifiers, among the sixty-eight who had become consultants, twenty-three held these posts in the region of their medical school, and nineteen of these had also held senior registrarships in the region of their medical school. Altogether, thirty-seven qualifiers had been senior registrars in the region of their medical school, and thirty-nine held consultant posts in the region where they had been senior registrars.

For the 1977 qualifiers, among forty-six who had become consultants, twenty held posts in the region of their medical school, and fifteen had also been senior registrars in the region of their medical school. Altogether, forty-two qualifiers had been senior registrars in the region of their medical school, and twenty-nine held consultant posts in the region where they had been senior registrars.

Table 13.11 shows that movement between regions during anaesthetics training was fairly typical of hospital specialties in general: anaesthetists appeared rather less likely than average to hold senior registrarships in the region of their medical school, and rather more likely to settle as consultants in the region of their senior registrarship; the 1977 respondents as a whole tended to stay closer to home than the 1974 respondents, but none of the differences was large.

Table 13.10 Location of senior registrar and consultant posts in anaesthetics in relation to medical school

Year of qualifying	*Senior registrar*	*Consultant*	*No. of respondents*	
1974	A	A	19	23 consultants in region of medical school
	B	A	3	
	?	A	1	
	A	B	6	
	B	B	20	incl. 2 with subsequent C
	?	B	1	
	B	C	18	incl. 1 with subsequent D
Total consultants			68	
	A	0	12	
	B	0	13	
	?	0	0	
Total senior registrars			93	
1977	A	A	15	20 consultants in region of medical school
	B	A	5	
	?	A	0	
	A	B	2	
	B	B	14	
	?	B	2	
	B	C	8	
Total consultants			46	
	A	0	25	
	B	0	45	
	?	0	3	
Total senior registrars			119	

Notes: A same region as medical school
B different region from medical school
C different region from senior registrarship
? region not stated
For London medical schools 'same region' equals Central London and the four Thames regions
Source: Parkhouse and Ellin 1990b

Table 13.11 Location of senior registrar and consultant posts in anaesthetics, and in all hospital specialties combined

Year of qualifying		*Senior registrar in region of medical school*	*Consultant in region of medical school*	*Consultant in region of senior registrar*
1974	Anaesthetics	40.7% (37 of 91)	33.8% (23 of 68)	59.1% (39 of 66)
	All hospital specialties	41.3% (237 of 574)	31.1% (127 of 409)	48.9% (171 of 350)
1977	Anaesthetics	36.8% (42 of 114)	43.5% (20 of 46)	65.9% (29 of 44)
	All hospital specialties	46.0% (271 of 589)	45.6% (87 of 191)	62.8% (108 of 172)

Notes: Percentages are of those with posts of known location
Locations refer to first substantive senior registrar and/or consultant post held
Source: Parkhouse and Ellin 1990b

Among the 1974 qualifiers from London medical schools, twenty-one had held senior registrarships in central London or one of the Thames regions, and nineteen in other regions of England. Twelve held consultant posts in London or a Thames region, fourteen in other English regions, and one in Wales. For the 1977 qualifiers from London medical schools, nineteen had held senior registrar posts in London or the Thames regions, twenty-six in other regions of England and two in locations that were not given. Seven had held consultant posts in London or a Thames region, and seven in other regions of England.

Looking at movement between UK countries, thirteen (14 per cent) of the 1974 qualifiers who had become substantive senior registrars in anaesthetics held these posts in a different country of the UK from that of their medical school. Twelve of these were Scottish graduates holding senior registrarships in England, and one a London graduate holding a senior registrarship in Scotland. Among those who had become consultants, nine (13 per cent) held their posts in a different country from that of their medical school; eight were Scottish graduates holding posts in England and one was a London graduate holding a post in Wales. Of all the graduates from Scottish medical schools who had become senior registrars in anaesthetics, 63 per cent held their posts in England; of those who had become consultants, 57 per cent held their posts in England.

The pattern among 1977 qualifiers was similar. Nineteen (16 per cent) senior registrars were working in a different UK country from that of their medical school; fifteen of these were Scottish graduates, of whom thirteen were in England, one in Wales, and one in Northern Ireland, where a subsequent consultant post was also held; three were Welsh graduates working in England, where one subsequently held a consultant post; one was an English graduate working in Scotland. Eleven doctors (24 per cent) held consultant posts in different UK countries from that of their medical school; nine of these were Scottish graduates of whom seven were working in England, one in Wales, and one in Northern Ireland where a senior registrarship had previously been held; one was a Welsh graduate working in England where again a senior registrarship had previously been held, and one was an English graduate working in Scotland. Of the Scottish graduates who had become senior registrars in anaesthetics, 65 per cent held their posts outside Scotland (57 per cent in England); of those who had become consultants, 69 per cent were working outside Scotland (54 per cent in England).

COMMENT

Over 40 per cent of those 1974 and 1977 qualifiers who became senior registrars in anaesthetics had begun their postgraduate experience in other specialties. This must add strength and breadth to anaesthetics. Other qualifiers who became senior registrars obtained experience in other specialties after entering anaesthetics straight from the pre-registration year, although only about 22 per cent of this group did so. Among the 1977 qualifiers, after nine years, 53 per cent of the direct entrants to the specialty had already become consultants, compared to 22 per cent of those who began in other specialties. For 1974 qualifiers after nine years, 23 per cent of those who began in other specialties had become consultants and 43 per cent of direct entrants, the latter figure supporting the generally more rapid progress of anaesthetics post-holders among 1977 qualifiers suggested by Table 13.5. But after thirteen years, 70 per cent of the 1974 qualifiers who went straight into anaesthetics had become consultants, compared to 78 per cent of those who began in other specialties. The consultant posts obtained included those with involvement with intensive therapy or pain relief, and the fact that various facets of the specialty appeal to doctors of different personality and background of training is clear from the comments of some respondents.

Proportionately fewer women than men who chose anaesthetics as a career soon after qualifying had become senior registrars or consultants within the time-span of these studies; but those women who had become senior registrars, from both cohorts, did so slightly more rapidly than the men. In England and Wales at 30 September 1986, thirty-two (8.0 per cent) of senior registrars in anaesthetics were part-time; thirty of these were women. Twenty-three (2.7 per cent) registrars in anaesthetics were part-time; twenty of these were women. These are perhaps surprisingly low numbers; they would seem to be consonant, however, with our observation that among all our 1974 and 1977 respondents, only thirteen women had held part-time posts on the way to becoming senior registrars or consultants, and the total number of part-time anaesthetics posts held by all the women respondents was quite small. This could well be determined by supply rather than demand; the frequent call for more part-time posts to be available, and with less patchiness and bureaucratic delay, is backed by many unhappy comments from individual women doctors. Anaesthetics as a career offers a variety of patterns of work and is in this respect at an advantage over some other specialties; domestic circumstances were frequently given as a factor of major importance in career choice, or change of choice, among women doctors opting for anaesthetics seven years after qualifying, that is including those who had changed their choice *to* anaesthetics since the pre-registration year (Parkhouse and Ellin 1988a). Very few women with the FFARCS were not working in anaesthetics when we heard from them in our latest surveys, and only seven were unemployed at those particular times.

14 Individual specialties

General practice

The analysis of the career paths followed by doctors during the years between leaving medical school and settling upon a career, as shown in previous chapters for anaesthetics and psychiatry, can be developed in various ways. In relation to general practice, we developed one type of career path analysis for doctors who qualified in 1974 (Parkhouse 1989a). For 1977 qualifiers, we carried out a more detailed analysis of progress in relation to general practice, for graduates from Scottish medical schools (Ellin and Parkhouse 1986).

THE 1974 QUALIFIERS

By 1987 a great deal of career information was available to us for doctors who qualified in 1974. Figure 14.1 shows what had happened to those doctors who gave general practice as their first choice of career at the time when they last replied to us. This diagram is compiled principally from information given in replies received in 1987. However, in some cases it was possible to include doctors who did not reply to us in 1987, because they were already known to be settled in general practice and because detailed of their previous career choices and progress were known from earlier replies.

It seemed interesting to know how many doctors' careers had been interrupted for various reasons — particularly in comparing men with women. For the purpose of this analysis, we regarded a gap of more than three months as a career break, when reasons were given or when details of jobs were otherwise fairly complete. In the great majority of cases the reasons for a career break were either clearly stated or were obvious, for example pregnancy or travel abroad. In a few cases it was possible to make a reasonable assumption about whether the reasons for a break were domestic or otherwise; any residual doubts were put among 'other/unknown' reasons.

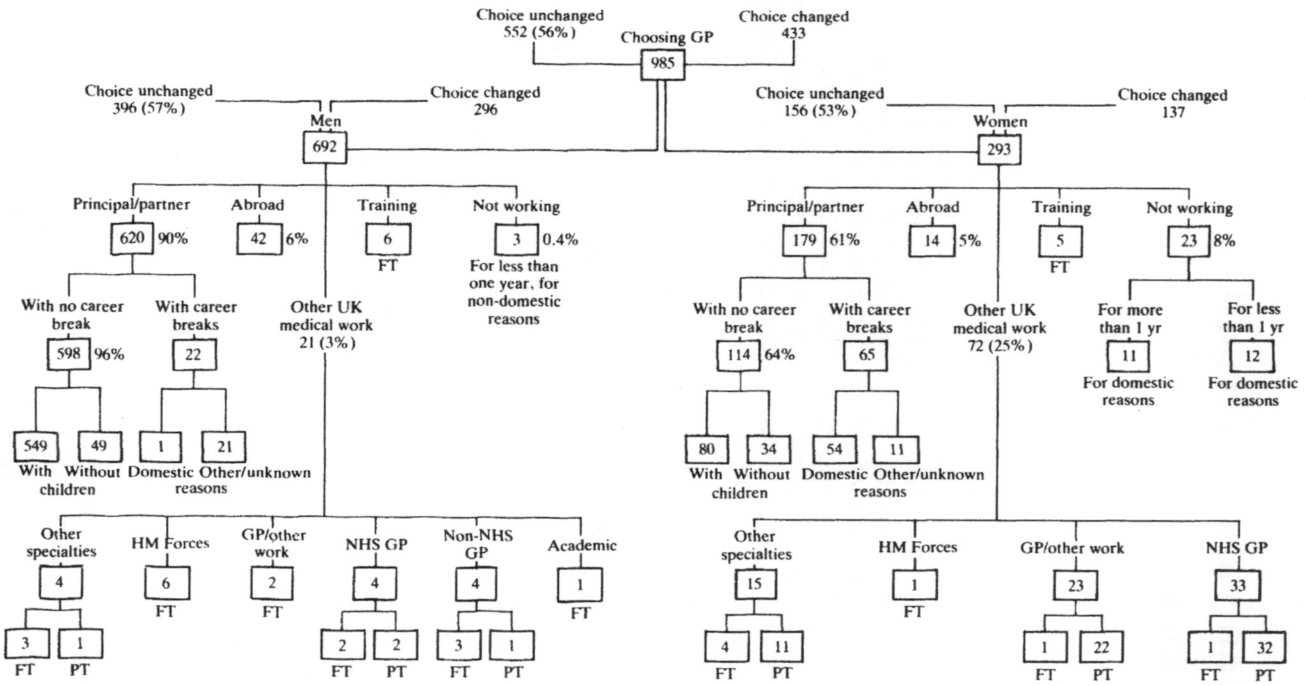

Figure 14.1 Career paths of 1974 qualifiers choosing general practice as a career
Source: Reproduced from *Update* (Parkhouse 1989a) by courtesy of the editor

We identified 985 doctors who gave general practice as their first choice of career when they last replied to us. Of these, 56 per cent had retained this as a constant first preference since the pre-registration year. In this respect, there was little difference between men (57 per cent) and women (53 per cent).

Concerning progress, 90 per cent of the 692 men were principals or partners, compared to 61 per cent of the 293 women (including salaried partners). Of these men 96 per cent had become principals without a significant break in their medical employment, which sometimes included experience abroad. Of the twenty-two with known gaps in working, only one specified domestic reasons. By contrast only 64 per cent of the women principals had worked without interruption, and where breaks had occurred they were due to domestic reasons, including moves with a husband, in 83 per cent of cases. Of the women who had become principals without a career break 70 per cent had children, but some of these doctors were working part-time; exact figures for this are hard to give since actual hours of commitment to general practice were often not stated.

For both men and women, general practice as a principal included clinical assistantships in a variety of hospital specialties.

Six men and five women were in general practice trainee, or SHO or registrar posts in hospital when they last replied. About the same proportions of men and women (5-6 per cent) were abroad. Three men and twenty-three women (8 per cent) were not working, the reasons given being domestic for all the women and otherwise for all three men. Eleven of the women had been out of work for more than one year at the time of their latest replies.

Twenty-one men (3 per cent) and seventy-two women (25 per cent) were in a variety of occupations not described above. The men included four in NHS general practice as locums or assistants, four in private general practice, one in an academic general practice appointment, two combining non-principal general practice work with other medical work, six in the Armed Forces and four in other specialties. Four of these twenty-one men were part-time. Among the women, thirty-three were in general practice as assistants, locums, or on the Women Doctors' Retainer Scheme, twenty-three were combining non-principal general practice work with other medical work, one was in the Armed Forces and fifteen were in other specialties, including community health, school or occupational medical services, and family planning; sixty-three of these seventy-two women (88 per cent) were part-time.

Looking at the experience of these doctors after twelve or

thirteen years from leaving medical school, it seems that general practice had a career to offer, in various ways, to nearly all of those who eventually decided they wanted to do it, and over half of them had always wanted to do it. Of the potential women general practitioners 10 per cent were not working at that stage, although many others were working part-time. It would be interesting for this, and for other reasons, to follow this cohort of doctors in another twelve or thirteen years to see what has become of them after twenty-five years as medical practitioners.

THE 1977 QUALIFIERS FROM SCOTTISH MEDICAL SCHOOLS

Up to September 1984, when this analysis was made, we had complete or partial career information about 598 doctors (95.1 per cent) who were identified by us as having qualified from Scottish medical schools in the calendar year 1977. Of the 598 respondents, 197 (32.9 per cent) gave general practice as their first choice of career at the pre-registration stage, either alone or tied with one or two other choices of career.

General practice was chosen by 114 men (30.9 per cent) and 83 women (36.2 per cent); its popularity varied between medical schools, from 42.9 per cent of corrected choices at Aberdeen to 24.3 per cent at Glasgow.

By August 1984 (roughly seven years after leaving medical school) 119 (60.4 per cent) of the 197 doctors who had chosen general practice within a year of qualifying were known to be, or to have been, principals in general practice (including partners with a limited commitment). This number included five doctors working in civilian general practice or family practice abroad, and two working as general practitioners in the Armed Forces (one of whom was abroad); it also included six doctors who had already left general practice and who were working in another specialty at the time of their last reply to us, and three who were already known to have moved from one general practice to another. There were a further twelve doctors for whom our records were insufficiently complete to know whether or not they had become principals by August 1984.

Only 35 of the 83 women choosing general practice (42.2 per cent) had become principals by August 1984, compared to 84 of 114 men (73.7 per cent). From Aberdeen medical school only two of the sixteen women choosing general practice (12.5 per cent) had become principals, the range of percentages of women doctors from the other three Scottish medical schools being from

45.5 to 57.9 per cent. This was a major reason for a lower overall 'achievement' rate for Aberdeen graduates of both sexes (53.5 per cent) compared to the other three schools (e.g. 66.7 per cent for Dundee).

Among the thirty-four graduates who had tied general practice with another first choice of career, only 35.3 per cent were known to have become principals by August 1984, compared to 65.6 per cent of those who gave general practice as an untied first choice. Furthermore, of respondents who at the pre-registration stage had made up their minds about their career choice 'definitely', 77.8 per cent were known to have become principals by August 1984, compared to only 53.8 per cent of those in the 'probably' or 'not really' groups.

For doctors who chose general practice *and* became principals by August 1984 the rate of progress showed some interesting features. For example 76.2 per cent of those 'definitely' choosing general practice had already become principals, compared to 46.8 per cent of those who had been less certain. During the six-month period between three and three and a half years following the start of the first post-registration appointment, the proportion of men becoming principals jumped from 16.7 to 65.5 per cent, while the corresponding proportion of women changed only from 8.6 to 37.1 per cent. During the following six-month period, however, the proportion of women become principals rose to 62.9 per cent.

It is interesting to note that in this group of doctors choosing general practice as a career there were two who went straight into general practice as principals immediately after the pre-registration year and two others who became GPs (one in the Armed Forces) during the following six-month period.

Other qualifiers entering general practice

In addition to the doctors who gave general practice as a first choice of career at the pre-registration stage, there were seventy-eight other respondents among Scottish qualifiers of 1977 who had become principals by August 1984. Of these, fifty-seven had given a different career choice from general practice in 1978, and twenty-one had not replied to our questionnaire at that time so that their career choice in 1978 is not known to us. Six doctors among the seventy-eight were working abroad in civilian general practice or family practice, and six were doing general practice in the Armed Forces (including one abroad).

Among those doctors whose career choice in 1978 was known

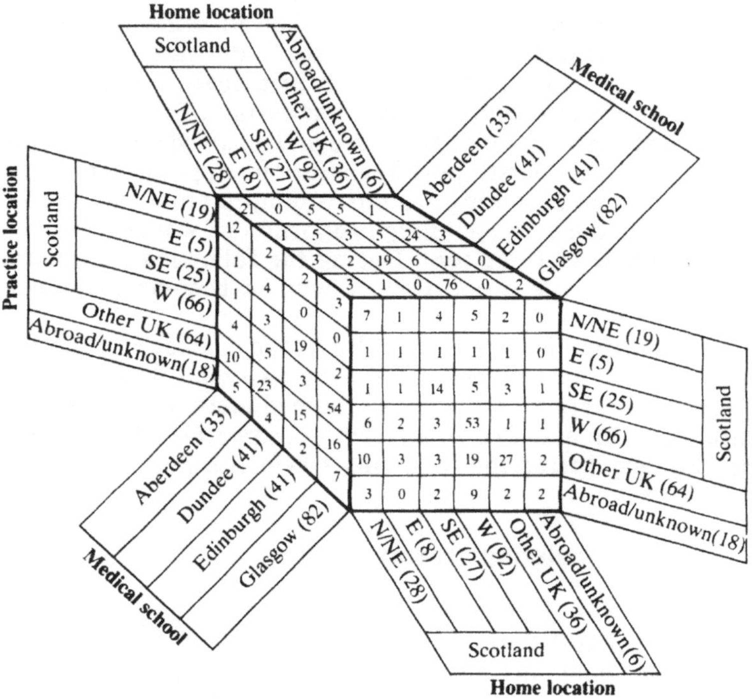

Figure 14.2 Qualifiers from Scottish medical schools in 1977 who became general practitioners by 1984: relationship between medical school, location of family home and location of general practice. Numbers of doctors with row and column totals in brackets

not to be general practice, and who had become principals by August 1984, two became GPs in the Armed Forces immediately after the pre-registration year, and four more (including three in the Armed Forces) became GPs during the six months following the end of the pre-registration year. This tendency to relatively rapid entry into general practice was sustained over the following three years, so that altogether 28.1 per cent of this group had become principals within three years of the beginning of their post-registration experience, compared to 14.3 per cent of those doctors who had given general practice as a choice of career at the pre-registration stage. Altogether, entry into general practice was much more evenly spread over time than among those who chose general practice in 1978, with men and women gaining roughly equal proportions of general practice appointments during the period of time studied.

Location of practice and movement

Altogether 197 respondents had become principals by August 1984 — 32.9 per cent of the respondents for whom career information was available. For the individual Scottish medical schools the numbers becoming principals, and the percentage which this represents of the number of respondents with known career information, were:

Aberdeen	33	(34.4 per cent)
Dundee	41	(44.1 per cent)
Edinburgh	41	(29.3 per cent)
Glasgow	82	(30.5 per cent)

In the cubic diagram (Figure 14.2) the three presenting faces of the cube show the relationship between medical school, location of general practice and location of family home. In this analysis, northern Scotland includes the northern and southern Highlands, Orkney and Shetland and the Western Isles.

Of the 197 respondents who had become principals, 58.4 per cent were working in Scotland. Most of the others were in England, but thirteen were working outside the UK and the location of five was unknown.

More than two-thirds of the respondents who had become GPs were working in the country of their family home. Of the 155 with family homes in Scotland, 68.4 per cent were practising in Scotland, with some regional differences. Fifty-three of the sixty-six (80.3 per cent) practitioners in the west of Scotland had family homes in that region, while only fourteen of the twenty-five working in the Edinburgh region (Lothian, Borders and Fife), six of the twelve working in the Grampian region and one of the five in Tayside came from homes in the corresponding parts of the country.

Proportionately much larger numbers of graduates from Aberdeen (39.3 per cent), Dundee (63.4 per cent) and Edinburgh (41.5 per cent) were practising outside Scotland than from Glasgow (25.6 per cent). Overall, 44.7 per cent of general practice respondents were practising in the Scottish 'region' of their medical school, with a wide range from 65.9 per cent of Glasgow medical school respondents in the west of Scotland to only 9.8 per cent of Dundee respondents in Tayside.

Of the respondents who became GPs, 118 (59.9 per cent) had attended a medical school in the 'region' of their family home. There were, however, considerable differences in this respect between the individual medical schools. Of the eight-two Glasgow medical school respondents, all but two were known to be from family homes in Scotland, and the location of one person's family home was unknown; seventy-six (92.7 per cent) were from family homes in the west of Scotland. At the other extreme, only five of the Dundee medical school respondents (12.2 per cent) were from homes in Tayside, and twenty-two — more than half their number — came from homes in the northern regions of England. Of the Aberdeen respondents 54.4 per cent were from family homes in the Grampian region, while 46.3 per cent of the Edinburgh respondents were from homes in Lothian, the Borders and Fife.

Taking all these factors together, seventy-one respondents who had become principals in general practice (36.0 per cent) had a family home, a medical school and a practice in the same 'region' of Scotland.

Doctors who had not become general practitioners by August 1984

Apart from the twelve doctors for whom, as noted above, we had insufficient data, sixty-six (33.5 per cent) of the 197 who had chosen general practice in 1978 were known not to have become principals by August 1984. We had adequate career data for sixty-four of these doctors.

Among this group — all of whom had given general practice as their first choice of career at the pre-registration stage — 62.5 per cent of women respondents but only 37.5 per cent of men still gave general practice as their first choice (including a few tied choices) when they replied to us in 1984: an overall percentage of 53.1 (thirty-four people).

Three women and one man were GP trainees at the time they replied to us in 1984; one man and one woman were locum GPs and one man was in a combined general practice/community medicine post on a locum basis. Of these seven doctors who were working in general practice at the time of their 1984 reply the three who were not currently trainees had previously completed a year as a GP trainee. Altogether, thirty-one of the sixty-four doctors in this group (48.4 per cent) had spent a continuous period of one year as a GP trainee. A small number of doctors had failed to complete a full year as a trainee, either because of domestic commitments or change to a different career.

Only two men and two women were currently in SHO posts so that altogether only a relatively small proportion of this group appeared still to be working towards a permanent career in general practice. One man was not working at the time of his 1984 reply. There were fourteen women doctors who were not working, plus three on the Women Doctors' Retainer Scheme. The reasons for not working were domestic in twelve cases – maternity, pregnancy, family commitments, young baby, and so on. In two cases movement was given as the reason for not working, but the unemployment was not necessarily unwelcome.

COMMENT

Generally speaking, the doctors concerned in this survey were sufficiently far advanced with their postgraduate training to be unaffected by the introduction of statutory vocational training requirements for general practice although, in fact, by the end of 1981 a considerable number of vocational training schemes were already operational in Scotland, mostly in the south-east. It is apparent from our data that, among 1977 qualifiers, the great majority of those who made a definite choice of general practice as a career at the pre-registration stage did not directly enter general practice, but tended to obtain three years of experience or thereabouts in hospital posts and in general practice before becoming a principal. On the other hand, doctors who did not choose general practice as a career on qualifying were more likely to enter general practice quickly, either when they made a career decision or when they decided, for various reasons, not to pursue an alternative career choice.

General practice was a popular career choice among Scottish

graduates in 1977, as it was throughout the UK, but for various reasons fewer than 60.0 per cent of the respondents in our survey who became GPs actually took up practices in Scotland. The different regions of Scotland showed varying degrees of 'self-containment', with quite striking variations in the numbers of doctors coming from family homes in the vicinity of the medical school and settling into a general practice in the same part of the country.

There were, seven years after qualifying, a substantial number of women doctors who were not working because of moves (which were often related to a husband's career) or domestic commitments. Most of these women doctors had obtained varying amounts of postgraduate training and experience, and many would very probably seek to re-enter medical employment at a later date.

15 Comments and opinions

In sending something in excess of 100,000 questionnaires to young doctors it is not surprising that we accumulated a large stock of comments. We made a point of emphasizing that all replies would be treated as strictly confidential, but it is nevertheless possible to capture the spirit of many of the views expressed, without their being attributable to any one person. We also met personally with some of our respondents, to discuss their problems and opinions, and in addition to our routine questionnaires we asked specifically at various times for views on the careers of women doctors (see Chapter 9) and on the quality and effectiveness of medical training.

Our first attempt at evaluating training and personal competence was made when we wrote to the 1974 qualifiers in 1983: 'What do young doctors think of their training and themselves?' (Parkhouse and Campbell 1984). Encouraged by this admittedly imperfect enquiry, we wrote again to the 1974 qualifiers in 1984, sending a very much more detailed questionnaire on the same theme. This also was an imperfect study, which nevertheless yielded useful information. On the basis of this experience, we included a supplementary questionnaire on evaluation (this time re-simplified) when we wrote to the 1980 qualifiers in 1985.

In each of these attempts to evaluate training and competence we identified five major elements of medical practice which we felt would be relevant to the work of all doctors, although in differing degrees, regardless of their specialty or type of work. These five elements were clinical/laboratory skills, communication, teaching, research, and administration/management.

THE 1974 QUALIFIERS IN 1983

For each of the five major elements of medical practice described above, we asked respondents to grade (1) importance

Table 15.1 Evaluation of training and competence (1974 qualifiers in 1983)[a]

	Meeting requirements 'very well'		*'Great need' for further competence or training*
	Undergraduate education	*Postgraduate training*	
Clinical/laboratory skills	45	60	16
Communication with patients and colleagues	19	46	12
Teaching	20	37	19
Research	9	39	33
Administration/management	1	16	36

Note: a Figures are percentages of those respondents who assigned major career importance to the element concerned (from 821 respondents for administration and management to 1,684 for communication)

Source: Adapted from Parkhouse and Campbell 1984 by permission from the *BMJ*

for their career, as 'not important', of 'minor importance', or of 'major importance'; (2) how well undergraduate and postgraduate training had met their requirements, as 'not at all', 'adequately', or 'very well'; (3) their need for further competence or training (or both), as 'no need', 'some need', or 'great need'.

It became clear from the replies that respondents had sometimes found it difficult to evaluate the first of these questions, because importance for their career could be taken to mean usefulness in passing examinations and obtaining promotion, or playing an important part in the work to be done when trained. Furthermore, if a respondent rated an element as being of little or no importance, it was not easy to interpret the significance of comments about whether training in that respect had been satisfactory: for example there were 533 respondents who rated research as unimportant, and 390 of these said that undergraduate training had not met their requirements. Bearing these problems in mind, the analysis of results was concentrated on respondents who assigned major career importance to the elements concerned. Table 15.1 presents results on this basis.

Clinical skills were regarded as of major career importance by over 86 per cent of all doctors except those in radiology (64 per cent), community medicine (63 per cent), and pathology (63 per cent). These findings may have been influenced by the fact that the wording of the question concentrated on clinical skills; in subsequent enquiries it was made more clear that both clinical and laboratory skills were considered relevant. Doctors with career choices for medicine and radiotherapy appeared most satisfied with their undergraduate training. In anaesthetics and radiology only about 20 per cent of respondents felt that the undergraduate course had met their requirements 'very well'. Postgraduate training, however, was rated highly by 74 per cent of anaesthetists and psychiatrists, but only by 39 per cent of respondents in community medicine. A 'great need' for further competence or training was most commonly felt by respondents in surgery (27 per cent).

Communication was thought to be of major career importance by 89 per cent of all respondents and, in general, postgraduate training was felt to have met requirements, fairly well. The range of difference among specialties was small, and only 12 per cent of those according major importance to communication felt a 'great need' for further competence or training.

Teaching was regarded as of major importance by only 30 per cent of respondents, varying from 28 per cent of those in general practice to 57 per cent in psychiatry. The general feeling was that undergraduate training had not met requirements: only 8 per cent of anaesthetists, for example, were very satisfied with this aspect of the undergraduate course. Although postgraduate training was more favourably regarded, only 15 per cent of respondents in community medicine thought it very satisfactory and, over all specialties, 19 per cent of respondents felt the need for further competence or training.

Research was regarded as of major importance by 55 per cent of respondents in medicine, but only 4 per cent of respondents in general practice, the average for all respondents being 24 per cent. Undergraduate training was thought to have been no help at all in research by 67 per cent of respondents. Respondents in community medicine were most likely to be very satisfied with what their present postgraduate training had offered in research (61 per cent) but altogether 33 per cent of respondents felt a 'great need' for further competence or training.

Administration and management was considered to be of major importance by 43 per cent of respondents overall, but the range was from 14 per cent in obstetrics and gynaecology to 50 per cent in general practice and 52 per cent in psychiatry. Very few doctors (0.6 per cent) felt that undergraduate training had met their requirements 'very well', while 93 per cent felt that it had not met their requirements at all. Those who considered that postgraduate training had served them well in regard to

Table 15.2 Views on clinical/laboratory skills (1974 qualifiers in 1984)[a]

	How it applies personally	*Usefulness in furthering career/passing exams, etc.*	*Importance for work of chosen specialty*	*How well it was tested by main postgraduate exam. (MRCP, FRCS, etc.)*	*Need for more*
Breadth of experience gained during training					
– within career specialty	64	72	84	38	
– outside career specialty (including hospital elements of vocational training)	45	45	54	26	
Present degree of					
– basic clinical competence (e.g. history taking, physical examination, etc.)	74	67	88	45	29
– sub-specialization (e.g. endocrinology, vascular surgery, etc.)	41	43	49	21	29

Note: a Figures are percentages of those respondents answering the relevant question who gave high or very high ratings

administration and management ranged from 0 per cent in paediatrics and obstetrics and gynaecology to 40 per cent in community medicine.

Among the general comments made by respondents, it was interesting that the enquiry brought to light some wide differences of opinion about what is to be expected from training and about the importance — or perhaps the inadvisability — of admitting imperfection. For example comments ranged from the view that anyone who did not feel completely competent at the end of postgraduate training 'should be shot', to the more commonly expressed view that only an intolerably arrogant person would claim to have no professional weaknesses or deficiencies.

THE 1974 QUALIFIERS IN 1984

For this more detailed enquiry the five main elements of medical practice were each subdivided, as shown in the tables, and respondents were asked to distinguish between the *importance* of an element or sub-element for the actual work of their chosen specialty, and its *usefulness* in furthering their career, passing examinations, etc. Some supplementary questions were also asked, and generous space was allowed for comment.

Clinical/laboratory skills

Respondents were asked to rate their experience to date (ten years after qualifying) within their chosen specialty and outside their chosen specialty (see Table 15.2). They were also asked to rate their competence in the general work of their chosen specialty, and also in regard to sub-specialization, for example for a physician, in cardiology, endocrinology, etc., and for an anaesthetist, in neurosurgical anaesthesia, paediatric anaesthesia, etc. As well as making a judgement on the importance of these sub-elements in the work of their specialty, and their value for promotion, respondents were asked to estimate how well they had been tested by the main postgraduate examination of their specialty, and their need for more competence or training.

Respondents were asked to grade all their replies on a scale 0-4: 0 = none, 1 = low, 2 = moderate, 3 = high, 4 = very high/essential. The tables in this section show the percentages of respondents who answered the relevant question and who gave a rating of 3 or 4.

Table 15.3 Views on postgraduate training (1974 qualifiers in 1984)[a]

	Pre-reg. year	*SHO/ registrar period*	*GP trainee year*	*Senior registrarship*	*Other training*	*How well it was tested by main postgraduate exam. (MRCP, FRCS, etc.)*	*Need for more*
Content of training posts							
– Practical experience without supervision	55	76	78	86	68		
– Practical experience with supervision	55	58	46	38	50		
– Formal instruction and courses	9	31	43	30	45		
Contribution to development of competence							
– Knowledge ('knowing what to do')	59	80	70	79	64	64	39
– Ability ('being able to do it')	53	77	67	80	61	20	32
– Judgement ('deciding whether to do it or not')	34	68	73	86	61	35	34

Note: a Figures are percentages of those respondents answering the relevant question who gave high or very high ratings

Table 15.4 Views on communication and teaching (1974 qualifiers in 1984)[a]

	Ability	*Usefulness in furthering career/passing exams, etc.*	*Importance for work of chosen specialty*	*Need for more*
Communication				
– with patients and their relatives	84	37	91	29
– with medical colleagues	69	57	89	23
– with other health professionals (e.g nurses, administrators)	63	29	86	23
– with others (e.g. general public, media, industry)	28	18	46	23
Teaching				
– clinical/bedside	47	34	55	27
– seminar/small group	44	31	52	26
– formal/theoretical (e.g. lecturing)	29	28	39	24
– of patients, general public, etc. (health education)	49	26	74	35

Note: a Figures are percentages of those respondents answering the relevant question who gave high or very high ratings

Although 74 per cent of respondents rated their competence in their chosen specialty as high or very high and 64 per cent rated their experience in the same way, only 45 per cent thought highly or very highly of their experience outside the specialty of their choice, and only 41 per cent gave such ratings in relation to sub-specialization. Importance for the work of the specialty was rated more highly than usefulness for promotion in relation to all four sub-elements. Only 38 per cent of respondents felt that their experience in their specialty had been well or very well tested by their principal postgraduate examination, and only 26 per cent felt this in relation to experience outside their chosen specialty. Again, only 45 per cent felt that their basic competence in their chosen specialty had been well or very well tested by their principal examination, and 21 per cent felt that the examination had tested them well or very well in regard to sub-specialization. A high or very high need for further competence in the chosen specialty in general, or in sub-specialization, was felt by only 29 per cent of those who answered the question.

Table 15.3 shows in a similar fashion the responses to questions concerning the way in which various stages of postgraduate training had been of value, first in regard to the content of various training posts, and second, their contribution to the development of competence.

Over 50 per cent of respondents rated the pre-registration year highly or very highly in regard to its content of experience without supervision and experience with supervision, and also its contribution to knowledge (knowing what to do) and clinical ability (being able to do it). In terms of judgement (deciding whether to do it or not), however, the pre-registration year was less highly rated, and only 9 per cent of respondents who answered the question felt that its content was high or very high in regard to formal instruction. In fact, formal instruction was the most poorly rated of all sub-elements throughout all phases of training, including the general practice trainee year. The most highly rated elements (given as high or very high by 86 per cent of those who answered the question) were for experience without supervision and the development of judgement during the senior registrar period. Interestingly the need for more was rated highly or very highly by more respondents in relation to knowledge (39 per cent) than for judgement (34 per cent) or for ability (32 per cent). Conversely the major postgraduate examinations were thought to have tested knowledge well or very well by 64 per cent of respondents who answered the question, but judgement was thought to have been well or very well tested by only 35 per cent, and ability by only 20 per cent.

Communication

Table 15.4 shows that communication with patients and relatives was regarded as important or very important by 91 per cent of respondents who answered this question, and similarly personal ability was highly or very highly rated by 84 per cent. On the other hand, only 37 per cent of respondents felt that this aspect of communication was of high or very high *usefulness* in achieving promotion and passing examinations. Indeed communication with medical colleagues was considerably more highly rated in this respect. But this and communication with other health professionals was regarded as *important* or very important for the work of the chosen specialty by over 85 per cent of respondents, whereas communication with the public, the media, etc. was so regarded by less than 50 per cent.

The need for more competence or training in the art of communication was not on the whole highly rated in response to these questions. There were, however, a considerable number of comments about the importance of communication and deficiencies in the teaching of communication skills (Rhodes 1989c). Many doctors thought that the importance of communication skills had been undervalued in their training. There was criticism of the 'over-emphasis' on the importance of 'academic' medicine at the expense of the 'art — understanding and talking to patients'. One respondent (working in community medicine) wrote:

> A patient who is not well wishes to see a competent, caring doctor who can explain the problem and solution in comprehensible language. He does not want a boffin who is interested more in his HLA antigens than his person.

A female respondent noted:

> The art of communication with patients and colleagues is not really emphasized at undergraduate level . . . tends to be acquired, sometimes painfully and sometimes inadequately, by experience.

Failure to communicate effectively with medical colleagues and with other health workers was also noted by respondents, several of whom suggested that joint training with other health professionals would be helpful. Another wrote:

> Medical colleagues are the most difficult to communicate

with: this does require a special training.

Teaching

Not surprisingly, fewer respondents (only 29 per cent) rated their ability highly or very highly in relation to formal teaching than for small group teaching (44 per cent) or bedside teaching (47 per cent). Table 15.4 further shows that formal teaching was also regarded as less important for the work of respondents' chosen specialties, and of less value in achieving promotion, but altogether only just over half of the respondents who answered the question considered that bedside teaching was an important or very important part of their work, and only about a quarter of the respondents felt a great or very great need for more competence or training in any aspect of teaching, except to do with the teaching of patients and the public, and health education. This, also, was more commonly rated as an important or very important aspect of work than any other kind of teaching (by 74 per cent of respondents to the question).

Some specific questions concerning teaching were included in the questionnaire. For example 16.9 per cent indicated that they had personally received organized instruction in how to teach at some stage. In answer to the statement 'It is important to produce doctors who can teach', 82 per cent felt strongly or very strongly in agreement. To the statement 'Teaching is a gift which cannot be learned', only 14 per cent agreed strongly or very strongly. One-third (33 per cent) of respondents felt strongly or very strongly that teaching ability should count heavily towards appointments and promotions in general practice or for NHS consultant posts; 94 per cent felt strongly or very strongly that teaching ability should count heavily towards appointments and promotions to medical posts in universities.

Research

Respondents were asked to consider four sub-elements of research: the assessment of research, e.g. as reported by others in the medical journals; personal participation in research; personal publication of articles and/or obtaining of a higher degree; directing research, formulating projects and influencing research policy. In analysing the responses, a distinction was made between respondents who were known to hold an optional intercalated degree, respondents from the Oxford and Cambridge clinical medical schools, and others. The overall response rate to the 1984 questionnaire was 66.6 per cent. Based on the 1,481 replies received to relevant questions, 76 per cent of Oxbridge respondents, 86 per cent of those with optional intercalated degrees, and 61 per cent of other respondents indicated that they had at some time been personally involved in research.

Table 15.5 shows that in regard to each of the four sub-elements, Oxbridge graduates and holders of optional intercalated degrees more commonly gave high or very high ratings than did other respondents in regard to perceived importance for the actual work of their chosen specialties, and also for usefulness in gaining promotion. The differences between the three groups of respondents in their self-rating of the need for greater ability were much less marked, and this might accord with the fact that their respective starting-points of current ability, as shown in Table 15.6, were rated somewhat in relationship to importance and usefulness. What is most interesting from Table 15.6 is the low perception of ability, in all aspects of research, among women as compared to men except in the Oxbridge group.

The responses to three specific statements in the questionnaire are shown in Table 15.7. There were no significant differences between the three groups in their views on undergraduate research or NHS consultant appointments. On the importance of producing doctors with an understanding of research there was a significant difference (chi-square, $p<0.01$) between the Oxbridge graduates and those with no intercalated degrees.

Among the individual comments, from all three groups of qualifiers, forty-three respondents (2.9 per cent) mentioned having done an intercalated degree, of whom only five commented in a positive way. Eleven respondents mentioned undergraduate research projects, two mentioned research electives and thirty-four others noted some research involvement at the undergraduate stage without giving details. Five respondents mentioned undergraduate publications. No respondents went out of their way to comment favourably on research at the undergraduate level. One thought his intercalated degree 'worth while' but regarded research as a 'vastly overrated enterprise'. One felt that the majority of students do not benefit; another thought that research for undergraduates 'should be illegal'. Without being specifically related to the undergraduate period, the most frequent comments related to the excessive emphasis placed on research and publications in the race for promotion; this was referred to, often with considerable bitterness and cynicism, by 108 respondents (7.3 per cent). In more general

Table 15.5 Percentages of respondents rating each element highly or very highly (1974 qualifiers in 1984)

Elements	*Respondents*	*Usefulness*[a] *in furthering career/passing exams, etc.*	*Importance*[a] *for work of chosen specialty*	*Need for*[b] *more competence/training*
Assessing research, e.g. published papers	No intercalated degree	39	45	33
	Optional intercalated degree	50	61	34
	Oxbridge	54	62	34
Participating in research	No intercalated degree	44	38	34
	Optional intercalated degree	59	49	36
	Oxbridge	64	52	41
Publishing papers and/or obtaining a higher degree	No intercalated degree	47	34	33
	Optional intercalated degree	62	50	39
	Oxbridge	63	48	41
Directing research, formulating projects, influencing policy, etc.	No intercalated degree	30	31	32
	Optional intercalated degree	42	46	38
	Oxbridge	43	42	37

Notes: a The differences between the group with no intercalated degree, and the other two groups combined, are all significant (chi-square $p<0.01$)

b No significant differences except for publishing papers/obtaining higher degrees, between no intercalated degree group and other two groups combined ($p<0.05$)

Table 15.6 Self-evaluation of ability: percentages of respondents rating each element highly or very highly (1974 qualifiers in 1984)

Respondents		*Assessing research, e.g. published papers*	*Participating in research*	*Publishing papers and/or obtaining a higher degree*	*Directing research formulating projects, influencing policy, etc.*
No intercalated degree (A)	Men	28	26	24	15
	Women	12	11	11	3
Optional intercalated degree (B)	Men	49	42	36	22
	Women	19	19	14	2
Oxbridge (C)	Men	39	32	32	19
	Women	39	29	26	16
chi-square sexes A cf. B		$p<0.001$	$p<0.001$	$p<0.01$	$p<0.05$
combined A cf.B		$p<0.001$	$p<0.01$	$p<0.01$	$p<0.01$

Table 15.7 Percentages of respondents who agreed strongly or very strongly with three statements (1974 qualifiers in 1984)

	No intercalated degree			*Optional intercalated degree*			*Oxbridge*		
Statements	*men*	*women*	*total*	*men*	*women*	*total*	*men*	*women*	*total*
1 It is important to produce doctors with an understanding of research[a]	62	64	63	71	67	70	72	77	73
2 All undergraduate medical students should undertake a research project[b]	37	41	38	42	48	43	30	42	32
3 Research and publications should count strongly towards NHS consultant appointments[b]	20	18	19	26	19	25	18	35	21

Notes: a Statement 1 – no intercalated degree group cf. other two groups combined chi-square $p<0.01$
– no intercalated degree group cf. Oxbridge group $p<0.01$
– no intercalated degree group cf. optional intercalated degree group ns

b No significant difference for other two statements (sexes combined)

terms, 106 respondents (7.1 per cent) felt there was too much emphasis on research with 'too many noddy papers around' and the 'phoney idea that to be a good doctor you need to be good at research'. The unkindest comment was from a doctor who felt that full-time research had

> wasted a year of my life and taught me how to manipulate data (?dishonestly) to produce papers which produced research grants which brought glory to the head of the department.

On the other hand 101 respondents (6.8 per cent) referred to the importance of research and the need for better training and understanding:

> No one can justifiably claim to be interested and concerned in patient care unless they have an active interest in continuing enquiry in their field of practice.

Fifty-seven respondents (3.8 per cent) specifically referred to the importance of being able to understand and evaluate research rather than being personally involved in it.

Administration/management

Table 5.8 shows the percentages of respondents answering the relevant questions who gave high or very high ratings to the five sub-elements of administration/management given in the questionnaire (Parkhouse *et al.* 1988).

The rating of *ability* was generally low, especially in regard to management training and financial management. It is also noteworthy that such a low proportion of respondents gave a high or very high rating to their present 'ability' concerning *knowledge* of the health care system and NHS administration. In regard to all the elements except obtaining and giving management training, *importance* was rated quite highly, but *usefulness*, in terms of career progress, and the *need for more* competence and training were both given much lower ratings than importance.

Except in regard to personnel management, women doctors rated themselves much lower than men as regards *ability*. With regard to *importance, usefulness* and the *need for more* competence or training, there was little difference between men and women.

Table 15.8 Views on administration and management (1974 qualifiers in 1984)[a]

	Ability	*Usefulness for promotion*	*Importance for work of specialty*	*Need for more competence/ training*
Knowledge of health care system/NHS administration	20	26	58	34
Business management (in GP, hospital department, clinical unit, etc.)	24	37	69	45
Financial management/ health economics	17	24	55	38
Personnel management/ industrial relations	28	27	63	31
Obtaining and giving management training	6	15	30	25

Note: a Figures are percentages of those respondents answering the relevant question who gave high or very high ratings
Source: Adapted from Parkhouse *et al.* 1988

Only 8 per cent of women respondents, and 16 per cent of men, felt strongly or very strongly in favour of leaving health service administration to professional administrators. Only 33 per cent of women said they had been involved in administration/management, compared with 57 per cent of men.

Career specialty differences

For *knowledge of the health care system and NHS administration, ability* was rated low in obstetrics and gynaecology, paediatrics and anaesthesia (9 per cent: percentages are respondents giving high or very high ratings, unless otherwise stated) and much more highly in community medicine (35 per cent) as might perhaps be expected. The *importance* of this knowledge was assessed highly in paediatrics (79 per cent) and psychiatry (76 per cent), and much less highly in obstetrics and gynaecology (47 per cent) and anaesthetics (43 per cent). However, the *usefulness* of knowledge was poorly rated in surgery (16 per cent) and paediatrics (19 per cent) and more highly in obstetrics and gynaecology (32 per cent) and psychiatry (41 per cent). Again, community medicine gave the highest rating (59 per cent). The *need for more* knowledge was strongly felt in psychiatry (53 per cent) compared with general practice (25 per cent).

For *business management, ability* was rated low in obstetrics and gynaecology (9 per cent), anaesthetics (11 per cent), paediatrics (13 per cent), surgery (16 per cent), and medicine (17 per cent), and much more highly in general practice (33 per cent). Its *importance* was again highly regarded in general practice (87 per cent), and also in radiology (67 per cent) and pathology (60 per cent). But only 20 per cent of pathologists regarded its *usefulness* as high or very high, and only 13 per cent of radiologists. Ten radiologists (33 per cent) felt that it had no usefulness. The *need for more* competence was highly rated in pathology (51 per cent), general practice (48 per cent), radiology (47 per cent), medicine (45 per cent), anaesthetics (40 per cent) and in psychiatry and community medicine (39 per cent).

For *financial management, ability* was poorly rated in all specialties, the highest self-assessments being in community medicine (26 per cent) and general practice (23 per cent). Its *importance* was most highly rated in general practice (70 per cent) and community medicine (57 per cent), and was considered lowest in surgery (29 per cent) and obstetrics and gynaecology (27 per cent). Interestingly the twenty-six respondents who were grouped as being in 'other medical' occupations (which includes medical work outside the NHS) gave a high rating to the importance of financial management and health economics (65 per cent). The *usefulness* of competence in financial management was most highly rated in general practice and community medicine, in contrast to surgery, paediatrics and pathology. In fact, in surgery 35 per cent of respondents rated its usefulness for career progress as nil. The *need for more* competence was most strongly felt in community medicine and pathology (44 per cent), psychiatry (43 per cent) and general practice (40 per cent).

In *personnel management*, 41 per cent and 40 per cent of respondents in obstetrics and gynaecology and anaesthetics respectively, 39 per cent of those in radiology and 31 per cent in surgery felt they had little or no *ability*, but this applied also to 49 per cent of paediatricians. *Importance* of personnel management was generally rated highly, especially in psychiatry (74 per cent), pathology (71 per cent) and general practice (69 per cent), but less so in obstetrics and gynaecology (53 per cent), anaesthetics (51 per cent) and surgery (50 per cent). Despite this perceived importance, only 31 per cent of respondents in pathology rated its *usefulness* as high or very high, and it was considered to have no usefulness by 37 per cent of those in radiology, and 30 per cent in paediatrics. Fewer than 50 per cent of respondents in any specialty felt a high or very high *need for more* competence; only 27 per cent in general practice and surgery, and 31 per cent in anaesthesia.

Ability in regard to *management training* was uniformly considered to be poor. Its *importance* was most highly felt in psychiatry (52 per cent) and community medicine (45 per cent), and least in obstetrics and gynaecology (18 per cent) and paediatrics (15 per cent). *Usefulness* was highly or very highly rated by 25 per cent or fewer of respondents in all specialties except for community medicine (41 per cent), and indeed only by 13 per cent in general practice. In surgery, 70 per cent of respondents felt that obtaining and giving management training had little or no usefulness. The *need for more* management training was felt to be highest in psychiatry (41 per cent), paediatrics, medicine and community medicine (32 per cent). The need was least strongly felt in general practice (20 per cent) and obstetrics and gynaecology (18 per cent).

The feeling that *doctors should run the NHS* was highest in surgery (42 per cent), pathology (41 per cent) and general practice (39 per cent). It was lowest in community medicine (24 per cent) and psychiatry (23 per cent). All specialties strongly favoured the *participation of doctors*. Those most inclined *to leave administration to professional administrators* were in obstetrics and gynaecology (24 per cent), and — surgery (21 per cent)! The least inclined were in community medicine and pathology (7 per cent).

Concerning the inclusion of management training at *undergraduate* level, the highest proportion of zero ratings, that is the strongest feeling against this was in obstetrics and gynaecology and pathology. Management training for doctors in *conjunction with other health professionals* was most strongly favoured in psychiatry (76 per cent) and least strongly in surgery (50 per cent).

Medical school differences

Knowledge of the health care system was clearly considered *important* by respondents from some medical schools (St George's 80 per cent, Liverpool 75 per cent) and less so by others (Dundee 38 per cent, Oxford 39 per cent, Guy's 41 per cent: percentages are respondents giving high or very high ratings, unless otherwise stated). The rating of importance was not fully echoed, however, by the perceived *need for more* competence (Oxford 21 per cent, St George's 50 per cent).

Ability in *business management* was felt to be reasonably high from the Oxford and Westminster medical schools (39 per cent), the lowest ratings being from Bristol and Sheffield (15 per cent). Its *importance* was highly rated by respondents from Leeds (82 per cent) and Wales (80 per cent).

Ability in *financial management* was felt to be very low by some graduates (St Thomas' and Aberdeen 7 per cent) but higher by others (Leeds 29 per cent). Its *importance* was highly rated by Welsh graduates (79 per cent) and given the lowest rating by those from Bristol (46 per cent) and Guy's (43 per cent).

Ability in *personnel management* was most poorly rated by Sheffield graduates (10 per cent) and most highly by those from Westminster (40 per cent). Its *usefulness* in terms of career progress was felt to be considerable by Royal Free Hospital and Aberdeen graduates (40 per cent) and very much less so by others (Liverpool 16 per cent). The *need for more* competence was rated lowest by Bristol graduates (17 per cent) and highest by Westminster graduates (46 per cent) who also gave the highest rating for their present ability.

The *importance* of *management training* was given most prominence by graduates from Dundee and Westminster (41 per cent) and least by Sheffield graduates (18 per cent). *Usefulness* was generally considered to be small, the highest rating coming from Aberdeen (26 per cent) and the lowest from Sheffield and Bristol (8 per cent). The *need for more* management training was most strongly felt among Manchester (36 per cent), St George's (33 per cent), Dundee and St Thomas' (32 per cent) and St Mary's (31 per cent) graduates, and least strongly from Birmingham (15 per cent) and Bristol (11 per cent).

The feeling that *doctors should run the NHS* emerged strongly among graduates from Wales and St Mary's (49 per cent) compared with those from Dundee and Middlesex (23 per cent). *Participation* was strongly favoured among all graduates (Aberdeen 100 per cent). The inclination to *leave administration to professional administrators* was highest among St George's graduates (27 per cent) and lowest from Westminster (out of thirty-six respondents: 3 per cent). Opinions appeared to vary considerably regarding the *value of management training at undergraduate level* (Charing Cross 37 per cent; Manchester 35 per cent; Middlesex 8 per cent). Those most strongly in favour of *training in conjunction with other health professionals* were from Westminster (67 per cent), University College Hospital (64 per cent), Royal Free (63 per cent) and Liverpool and Manchester (62 per cent). Those least in favour were from Sheffield (40 per cent), Oxford (39 per cent) and St Thomas' (38 per cent).

Comments

The largest number of individual comments referred to the need for doctors to participate actively in NHS management, and the dangers of not doing so (forty-seven: numbers in parentheses refer to the number of individual comments relating to each topic).

> Consultants in the NHS have let the system fall into its present all-time low because of their lack of interest in the service, their juniors or people working with them. And *now* they complain of the administration.

> Doctors at present are too lax and imagine that administrators have patients' and doctors' best interests at heart . . . They are merely concerned with balancing the books and blow the medical consequences.

> Most doctors have little idea how the NHS is managed, yet make many demands of the system — they are surprised and angry when they don't get what they want.

> Unless doctors are involved strongly in the running of the NHS the present shambles and low morale will get worse.

This was coupled with a variety of thoughts about the precise role of the doctor in this context. For example, a common view (twenty) was that doctors should be responsible for broad policy decisions and overall management control, while leaving day-to-day implementation of policy to professional administrators.

> Doctors should administrate with the help of professional administrators.

> Certain aspects of administration, e.g. salaries, finance (some aspects), holidays, etc., are far better left in the hands of professional administrators whereas others, e.g. planning, new developments, clinical services, should be managed by doctors.

One of the principal reasons for these views was the feeling that only a doctor has the necessary understanding of health problems and patient management to be able to make sensible decisions about NHS policies and priorities (twenty).

> Doctors *must* run the NHS (two).
>
> Non-medical managers simply will not understand what health care is necessary. If they are in control, then clinical care will be effectively dictated by people who do not have the ability to comprehend it.
>
> Until doctors are taught management principles so they can converse sensibly with professional administrators, thus ensuring that good management includes sensible clinical decisions, the NHS will continue to waste more money than it actually makes use of.

The present failures of communication and understanding in administration were a cause of concern:

> I find that junior hospital doctors are ignorant of NHS management, and that most administrators are (1) inaccessible, (2) unaware of the problems involved with running the more practical aspects of a ward/unit. I would welcome the opportunity to meet administrators — I don't think they know what my job actually involves, and most don't seem to be very interested. I have little idea what theirs involves, but would like to know.

There were also clearly some worries about the poor quality of NHS administration (eleven).

> One problem with the NHS is the explosion in numbers of administrators of low ability.

There was a feeling that doctors could, given the right conditions, do a better job than administrators in this respect (thirteen).

> Doctors are more likely to gain insight into problems experienced by managers than *vice versa*.

Several respondents commented, however, that doctors generally do not have sufficient time for serious involvement in management (ten), that it might be better to use trained administrators to represent doctors' interests (one), and to leave medical administrative involvement to senior doctors who are in a position to shed *some* of their clinical commitments, but not all.

> The problem is that doctors are only better than administrators while they are practising — if they have to give up their medical practice to administer we are no better off.

Some respondents made a plea for 'less administration in the NHS' (six) but some made the point that it is necessary to distinguish clearly between management and administration (six) and pointed out that it is *management* skills which are needed from doctors (three). Somewhat in contrast to the above comments were feelings that doctors do not on the whole make good administrators (fourteen).

> Probably the best comment on management in a financial sense, from a bank manager (admitting to a generalization): 'doctors are babes in arms when it comes to financial management of personal and practice affairs'.

> Good clinicians, in general, do not make good administrators.

Two respondents expressed the view that doctors should not 'top the hierarchy'.

A few respondents felt no need for administrative skills, because they had only a relatively small part-time clinical commitment (two), or were generally unenthusiastic about management and administration (six): 'please, no management training' (one). Several respondents stressed the need for *competent* people in administration and management (seven), whether doctors or not.

> If the management of the various Royal Colleges, the BMA and GMC are anything to go by, do not let the over-inflated, the narrow-minded or those tired of, or incompetent at, clinical medicine run the NHS. They took five to six years to train as doctors: how long do ICI, Shell etc. take to train their senior management?

Two respondents specifically referred to the importance of consumer involvement and the need for an 'open attitude' on the part of doctors:

> It amazed me when I joined various committees how genuinely naive and/or narrowly focused many of my consultant colleagues are — especially true of surgeons who seem to live in a black box immune from wishing to face up to social/economic and political realities of the NHS at present.

The importance of attitudes (and prejudices persisting or developing during postgraduate training) is obvious in this context.

> The most important question, sadly, is usefulness in furthering one's career which is virtually zero — usual middle-class prejudice against 'trouble makers' who are interested enough to participate in management as a junior doctor.

Four respondents were enthusiastic about what they saw as the advantages of the 'medical superintendent', and three of these respondents had personal experience of alternative health care systems abroad.

Management training was seen as a major omission from medical education and training by twenty-seven respondents.

> Lack of adequate training has been the most serious deficiency of my undergraduate and postgraduate education.

Some comments voiced a desire to see management training included in the undergraduate curriculum (twelve), but others felt that it was not advisable or useful at this stage.

> I feel it would be treated by students as not part of becoming a doctor, rather as we as students sadly rejected attempts to teach us statistics!

Its importance in postgraduate training was specifically referred to on twenty-two occasions. Five respondents commented on the value of courses they had attended, but four others doubted the usefulness of management training. Some wished to see it provided only for some doctors (eight) or for 'those interested' (five).

> Management/administration training should be extensively available to those committed or interested in this field, and they should be encouraged. For the average clinician, this

Table 15.9 Personal learning (1974 qualifiers in 1984)[a]

	Under-graduate education	*Intercalated degree*	*Pre-registration year*	*Post-graduate training*	*Academic experience*	*Feedback from others*	*Courses*	*Personality*	*Other*
Administration/ management	1	1	4	16	11	18	12	30	17
Teaching	16	3	9	31	27	38	13	42	14
Research	4	13	1	15	27	12	6	21	9
Communication	14	3	39	48	23	37	12	64	27
Clinical/ laboratory skills	43	9	61	64	27	24	16	35	13

Note: a Percentages of all respondents giving high or very high ratings

> field had little relevance to day-to-day work and 'blanket' training is wasteful.

The different needs of different specialties were referred to in relation to pathology (three), geriatrics, accident and emergency, community medicine, and psychiatry (five).

> In many ways I was naive and unprepared for the amount of administration involved in my post. This may be most applicable to psychiatry, which is under-resourced and under-financed, with high government and society expectations.

The importance of management in general practice was specifically referred to by twenty-six respondents.

Individual learning

The final section of the questionnaire attempted to find out how respondents felt that they had acquired their current competence in regard to the five elements of medical practice. For this broad, general enquiry, Table 15.9 shows the percentages of all respondents who gave high or very high ratings under each of the headings.

From these responses, undergraduate medical education appeared to have made little contribution to competence except in relation to clinical and laboratory skills, where its importance was still outweighed, perhaps not surprisingly, by the pre-registration year and postgraduate medical training. Few respondents rated specific courses highly or very highly in contributing to their competence, and although academic postgraduate experience was regarded as having made a high or very high contribution to research competence by 27 per cent of respondents, this was not very much higher than the significance attached to personality. As far as teaching was concerned, academic postgraduate experience was less often regarded as important or very important in contributing to competence than postgraduate medical training or feedback from students and self-learning. For the acquisition of communication skills, by far the most important factor emerged as the respondent's own personality, which was regarded as highly or very highly important by 64 per cent of respondents. Other experience, for example work abroad and non-medical activities, was seen to have made a greater contribution to communication skills than to

Table 15.10 Percentage of respondents answering question giving value 3 or 4 (1980 qualifiers in 1985)

		Usefulness of training and other experiences in developing ability			*Importance for*	
	Ability	*undergraduate education*	*postgraduate training*	*other experience*	*promotion etc.*	*work of specialty*
Clinical/laboratory skills	88	24	80	32*	59	89
Communication with						
– patients and relatives	91	14	60	57*	34	88
– doctors/nurses, etc.	87	15	58	40*	67	83
– others	73*	8*	37*	43*	37*	58*
Teaching						
– formal	28	15	29	22*	20	27
– informal/bedside, etc.	57	19	41	24*	19	45
Research						
– interpretation of data	28	22	25	20*	36	35
– personal involvement	21	12	20	17*	51	23
– planning and supervision	17	7	14	15*	39	24
Management						
– department/unit practice organization	34	1	34	26*	43	71
– understanding of health economics	19	3	19	21*	19	41
– policy-making, via committees, etc.	12	1	12	19*	24	38
– other	18*	1*	14*	17*	26*	27*

Note: * Question not answered by 1,000 (39%) or more respondents, all other questions answered by at least 87% of respondents

other elements. Feedback from others appeared to have made its greatest contribution towards ability in respect of teaching and communication.

THE 1980 QUALIFIERS IN 1985

The questionnaire was simpler than the 1984 questionnaire sent to 1974 qualifiers, and since the breakdown into sub-elements was somewhat different, the results are not always directly comparable. Respondents were again asked to grade their replies from 0 to 4, and Table 15.10 shows the percentages of those respondents answering each relevant question who gave ratings of 3 or 4. Some questions, particularly those relating to the value of 'other' experience, were left unanswered by considerable numbers of respondents. Where questions were not answered by 1,000 (39 per cent) or more respondents this is indicated in the table by an asterisk (*). All questions not so indicated were answered by at least 87 per cent of respondents.

Generally speaking, the findings are not inconsistent with the previous studies reported above. The low ratings assigned to the undergraduate course in regard to communication skills and understanding of management are again notable. In looking at management/administration generally, the 1980 qualifiers appeared to think slightly more highly of their ability in departmental organization, etc., and of its importance. They were rather less convinced of the importance of health economics, either for obtaining promotion or for the work of their chosen specialties. Again, men tended to rate their ability considerably more highly than women. In terms of perceived importance in relation to work to be done when trained, it is interesting to see that departmental or unit management, and practice organization was rated as of great or very great importance by almost as many respondents (71 per cent) as were clinical skills (89 per cent) and communication with patients, relatives and colleagues (over 80 per cent), and far more often than teaching or research.

MEETINGS WITH RESPONDENTS AND GENERAL COMMENTS

The informal meetings that took place with small groups of respondents at the NHS Training and Studies Centre in Harrogate (in 1984 and 1985) included discussion sessions which focused on three main topics: the career structure and postgraduate training, the role of counselling in career development, and the role of doctors in management. The ideas which emerged were not new; they were a cry from the heart from doctors involved in the process of postgraduate training about many of the problems and inadequacies that are well known. There was general agreement that specialization in medicine was becoming too rigid and too narrow, and that there must be greater flexibility in training. Also, in order to relate medical specialization to the efficient provision of health care to the community, the link between hospital medicine and general practice was seen to need considerable strengthening. With regard to the structure of postgraduate training, there was support for the idea of broader ranges of experience, with a system providing opportunity to obtain experience in a wide variety of specialties during the early postgraduate period. A possible means of achieving this would be to build upon the Todd Report's (1968) ideas for General Professional Training, by giving 'credits' for four- or six-month periods of experience. A sufficient number of 'credits' could be built up over perhaps a five-year period, so that time out could be allowed for domestic commitments and other activities not directly related to the immediate career path. The system should allow exit and entry to specialized pathways at various points, and while some aspects of training should be mandatory, much could be optional or selective. The increasing rigidity of the higher levels of postgraduate training, at the senior registrar stage, were regarded as a particularly undesirable development.

Careers counselling — as distinct from simply providing careers advice or information — emerged as an important topic during these meetings. Most of the participants took advantage of the presence of a professional counsellor at the first meeting, and several found this a soul-searching experience. The counsellor himself was considerably shaken by the unexpected amount of insecurity and anxiety to be found within a superficially successful and self-confident group of young professional people. The role of careers counselling in 'helping people to help themselves' (Milne 1984), through positive non-directive listening, was regarded as an important and seriously under-developed counter-weight to large-scale personnel planning.

The discussions about the participation of doctors in management took place against a background of considerable confusion regarding the development of management in the National Health Service, following the Griffiths Report (1983), and the place of the doctor in this development. There was a general view that doctors needed to know about management, but very little clarity on the question of how to go about it: a start should be made at the undergraduate level, with SHOs and registrars also being involved. One important feeling which was made clear was the need for collaboration with other health professionals, and for the doctor — particularly the consultant — to learn to participate co-operatively and non-autocratically.

These discussions with respondents thus underlined many of the views expressed in questionnaire replies and described in the preceding sections of this chapter. Very many written comments over the years gave evidence of strong feelings about the problems of the hospital career structure and the inimical attitudes in hospital medicine which lead many young doctors to turn towards an alternative career such as general practice:

> In pursuance of hospital medicine one has to make many sacrifices especially socially . . .

> *Ideally* I would have liked to pursue surgery but the hours etc. broke up my first marriage after eight years . . . I have now remarried and have two small children. I am just not prepared to spend 100 hours a week in a hospital . . . career prospects in surgery are atrocious.

> I have concluded that it is impossible for me to have a hospital career, whilst on one hand tired and disillusioned by long hours and relatively poor pay, and on the other having to work with poor facilities, dangerously low staffing levels and oppressed by inept bureaucracy.

> Starting to have doubts — my child doesn't know me. (Surgery)

> Consultants working themselves into early graves — plenty of guys seem keen to join them. I leave it to them. . . . General practice is a better way to practise *family* medicine than paediatrics.

> The difficulty of finding suitable training posts in the various specialties and the uncertainty of posts on completion of training — together with a fragmented life-style mitigates strongly against any hospital career.

> At the tender age of 27-28 one is becoming a 'has been' or 'also ran' if one has not progressed up the scale. . . . Surely the future of proper medicine in this country should be based

> on a stable background.

Many other comments indicated the lack of adequate careers counselling or guidance, and the sad effects of the rigidity of the system:

> No one had the concern or the courage to tell me that I wasn't going to succeed at a stage in my career when a change of specialty would have been more realistic and less painful.

> I note that interest and curiosity are no longer factors in choosing jobs which is why no doubt there is a shortage of doctors engaged in the exploration of the Antarctic but plenty to publish boring bloody statistics like these!

Conclusion

The doctors delivered into the world by the medical schools in 1983 opened their eyes on an arena of vast opportunity and baffling moral dilemma; a western world in which reaction had set in with some vengeance against the Beveridge era's faith in social security. It was a state in Britain not unlike that depicted by J.K. Galbraith in an address to Smith College in the USA where, in the interests of institutional truth, as he called it, you are required to believe,

> that, although we are still the world's richest country, we must tolerate in our great cities some of the world's most devastating and devastated slums. . . . More public housing, adequate welfare payments, adequately paid teachers, sufficient recreational facilities, more community action programmes would be, our wealth notwithstanding, too expensive. Additionally, such expenditure would . . . be damaging to the morals and economic morale of those so helped.
>
> (Galbraith 1989)

Thus newly qualified doctors in Britain faced the challenge of a two-nations kind of country in which social deprivation and consumerism existed side by side; a place of prosperity and hope for many, along with an uncomfortable amount of disillusioned, restive youth and cold, lonely old age; a nation with many one-parent families, two-family parents, and cohabiting professional couples with independent careers to pursue; an environment overwhelmed by technology and greed. There were significant differences of emphasis and degree in these respects from the world encountered by the medical graduates of the early 1970s. For instance, it is relevant that comparing 1979-83 with 1970-72, differences in Standardized Mortality Ratios between upper and lower social classes had widened, and there were large regional variations, despite the fact that overall mortality from all causes had declined (Balarajan *et al.* 1987). And by 1986 the proportions of patients having elective surgical operations performed privately varied from 31 per cent in two regions in London to 6 per cent in the north-east — a larger difference than in 1981 (Nicholl *et al.* 1989). Yet all in all, the not-so-brave new world of Britain was probably all the better for at least beginning to realize what was seriously amiss.

The practice of medicine was also dominated by new possibilities and concerns: not only by still more sophisticated means of investigation and treatment, amazing research, but also by complex ethical issues, financial stringency, litigation, AIDS, and anxiety for the future of the NHS. But within the structure of the system, and in its impact on postgraduate trainees, little had really changed except in the loss of some valuable flexibility. We began with reference to the Royal Commission on Medical Education in 1968, and its survey of medical students. Among those findings there is much in common with what we and others have found later among doctors. For example 13 per cent of final-year medical students in 1966 already had grave doubts about their choice of medicine as a career, and 40.8 per cent had slight doubts.

During the years covered by our studies, great opportunities have been lost in relation to medical careers, through inertia or complacency, the dominance of vested interests, fear of the unknown, lack of imagination or sheer incompetence. Overriding all this there has been, in the profession, and the governing bodies of its practitioners and their specialties, a preoccupation with high standards of clinical care, the importance of teaching and research, and with the doctor's independence of political domination in his or her legitimate work. These virtues, which are not unique to the UK, and also the muddles which doctors in this country have had wished upon them, are among the influences that have shaped the opinions and careers described in these pages.

Different interpretations and shades of emphasis can be read into the information and comment which we have been privileged to receive from so many young doctors. Most of this analytical thinking we leave to the reader. What the future holds for our respondents and their successors may perhaps be documented one day. This is just the story so far.

Appendix
Example of a 'standard' questionnaire

8	3					

Career preferences of 1983 graduates, follow-up inquiry 1986

All replies will be treated as strictly confidential. It would help us very much if you would please answer ALL questions. (See covering letter)

Name used professionally: ______________________

Maiden, married or former name, if applicable: ______________________

Current Address: ______________________

Date of Birth (please enter as shown) — Day Month Year — 8 [ ][ ][ ][ ][ ][ ]

FOR OFFICE USE

Sex: (Please ring appropriate number)

Male 1 Female 2 — 14 [ ]

Marital Status: (Please ring appropriate number)

Single 1 Married 2

*Other 3 — 15 [ ]

*Please specify ______________________

How many children do you have? (Please enter number in box) — 16 [ ]

Age of youngest child (in years) — 17 [ ][ ]

Since the beginning of 19 which postgraduate examinations have you passed?

(Please include Pt 1, Primary etc and give year)

____

____

____

____

FOR OFFICE USE

19 [ ][ ][ ]

22 [ ][ ][ ]

25 [ ][ ][ ]

Have you made up your mind about your choice of final career? (Please ring appropriate number)

Definitely 1 Probably 2

Not Really 3 — 28 [ ]

What is your career choice? List up to three choices in order of preference. Bracket together any choices that are equal. You can be as specific, or as general as you like.

1st ______________________ 29 [ ][ ][ ]

2nd ______________________ 32 [ ][ ][ ]

3rd ______________________ 35 [ ][ ][ ]

[ ]

Apart from temporary visits abroad, do you intend to practise in the United Kingdom? (Please ring appropriate number)

FOR OFFICE USE

Definitely Yes 1 Definitely No 2

Probably Yes 3 Probably No 4 — 39 [ ]

Undecided 5

Which of the following factors have been important in influencing your choice of career? For each one please enter the appropriate number in the box, using the following coding:

0 Not important 1 Minor importance

2 Major importance

A	Domestic circumstances	[ ]	40
B	Financial circumstances	[ ]	41
C	Knowledge of promotion/career prospects and difficulties	[ ]	42
D	Appraisal of your aptitudes and abilities	[ ]	43
E	Advice from others	[ ]	44
F	Experience of your chosen subject as an undergraduate	[ ]	45
G	Contact with a particular teacher/department	[ ]	46
H	Inclinations before entering medical school	[ ]	47
I	Additional experience of your **previous** choice of career	[ ]	48
J	Additional experience of your **present** choice of career	[ ]	49
K	Other reasons*	[ ]	50

* Please specify ______________________

____

____

____

____

Please list all POSTS held and indicate periods of UNEMPLOYMENT since the beginning of 19   ending with your PRESENT JOB(S)

If any of the jobs listed was:

Within the Armed Forces, please indicate by ticking column 2;
Part of GP vocational training, please indicate in column 4 using the following coding:
A = a formal scheme   B = a self-arranged scheme;
Part of a hospital rotation scheme, please indicate by ticking column 5;
Part-time, please give the number of weekly sessions worked in column 6.

1 Specialty	2 Armed Forces	3 Grade/Type of post (Please state if locum)	4 GP Voc.	5 Hosp Rotn	6 Part-time Sessions	7 Dates From	To	8 Location (Town/City)
Present Job(s)								

If you are CURRENTLY UNEMPLOYED

(a) Please give the date when you became unemployed and the reason for your unemployment

Date: ____________________

Reason: ____________________

____

____

(b) Are you currently seeking employment? (Please ring appropriate number)

No 1   Yes, part-time 2

Yes, full-time 3

FOR OFFICE USE

51 ☐

52 ☐

53 ☐

FOR OFFICE USE

54
66
15
26
37
48
59
70

PLEASE RETURN THIS FORM IN THE PRE-PAID ENVELOPE TO: DR JAMES PARKHOUSE, MEDICAL CAREERS RESEARCH GROUP, CHURCHILL HOSPITAL, HEADINGTON, OXFORD OX3 7LJ

Bibliography

Publications arising from this research project on doctors' careers are marked with an asterisk (*). Not all of these are specifically referred to in the text of this book.

Abel-Smith, B. and Gales, K. (1964) 'Emigration of Doctors', *British Medical Journal* ii: 53.

Alexander, D.A. (1988) 'Loans for medical students', *British Medical Journal* 297: 1,561.

Allen, I. (1988) *Doctors and their Careers*, London: Policy Studies Institute.

Angold, A. (1979) in 'Who puts medical students off psychiatry?', a meeting of the Association of Psychiatrists in Training, held at the London Hospital Medical College on 6 February 1972, London: SK & F Publications.

Balarajan, R., Yuen, P. and Machin, D. (1987) 'Inequalities in health: changes in RHAs in the past decade', *British Medical Journal* 294: 1,561-4.

Beaumont, B. (1978) 'Training and careers of women doctors in the Thames regions', *British Medical Journal* i: 191-3.

Berliner, H. (1988) 'The female phenomenon', *Health Service Journal* 9 June: 650.

Bhate, S., Sagovsky, R. and Cox, J.L. (1986) 'Career survey of overseas psychiatrists successful in the MRC Psych examination', *Bulletin of the Royal College of Psychiatrists* 10: 121-3.

Birtchnell, J. (1987) 'Recruitment into psychiatry', *Society of Clinical Psychiatrists* SCP Report no. 14, Supplement to *British Journal of Clinical and Social Psychiatry* 5 (2).

Blalock, H.M. (1982) *Social Statistics* 2nd edn, London: McGraw-Hill, 396-412.

BMA (British Medical Association) Conference (1989) Report in *Guardian* 7 July.

Brook, P. (1976) 'Where do psychiatrists come from?', *British Journal of Psychiatry* 128: 313-17.

Clayden, A.D. and Parkhouse, J. (1971) 'Allocation of pre-registration posts', *British Journal of Medical Education* 5: 5-12.

— (1972) 'Promotion in the National Health Service and the effect of change', *British Journal of Medical Education* 6(1): 9-12.

Clayden, A.D., Knowelden, J. and Parkhouse, J. (1971) 'A "general professional training" inquiry', *Postgraduate Medical Journal* 47: 201-6.

Davison, R.H. (1962) 'Medical emigration to North America', *British Medical*

Journal i: 786-7.

Delamothe, T. (1988) 'Blood, sweat, and tiers', *British Medical Journal* 297: 756.

DHSS (Department of Health and Social Security) (1969) *The Responsibilities of the Consultant Grade*, Report of the Working Party appointed by the Minister of Health and the Secretary of State for Scotland (Godber Report), London: HMSO.

— (1976) Draft 'Women in Medicine: Improving Opportunities for Doctors with Domestic Commitments to practise in the NHS', JC63 1975-76, London: DHSS.

— (1978) *Medical Manpower – The Next Twenty Years*, London: HMSO.

— (1980) *Medical Manpower Steering Group Report*, London: DHSS.

— (1985) *Report of the Advisory Committee for Medical Manpower Planning*, London: DHSS.

— (1986) *Hospital Medical Staffing: Achieving a Balance*, London: DHSS.

— (1987a) 'Medical and dental staffing prospects in the NHS in England and Wales in 1986', Medical Manpower and Education Division, *Health Trends* 19(3): 1-8.

— (1987b) *Plan for Action – Hospital Medical Staffing: Achieving a Balance*, London: DHSS.

DoH (Department of Health) (1989) *Report of the Second Advisory Committee for Medical Manpower Planning*, London: Department of Health.

Doyal, L., Gee, F., Hunt, G., Mellor, J. and Pennell, I. (1980) *Migrant Workers in the NHS*, London: Polytechnic of North London.

Dunlop, D. (1975) Reply on behalf of the honorary medical graduates, *University of Nottingham Gazette*, September, 86: 2,079.

Eaton, D.G. and Thong, Y.H. (1985) 'The Bachelor of Medical Science research degree as a start for clinician-scientists', *Medical Education* 19: 445-51.

Egerton, E.A. (1979) 'Medical undergraduate career preference enquiry', *Ulster Medical Journal* 48: 43-61.

— (1980) 'Survey of Queen's University medical graduates', *Ulster Medical Journal* 49: 112-25.

— (1985) 'Choice of career of doctors who graduated from Queen's University, Belfast in 1977', Northern Ireland Council for Postgraduate Medical Education, Belfast, Northern Ireland, *Medical Education* 19: 131-7.

— (1987) 'Women in medicine', in R.D. Osborne, R.J. Cormack and R.L. Miller (eds) *Education and Policy in Northern Ireland*, London: Policy Research Institute, 151-66.

*Ellin, D.J. and Parkhouse, J. (1986) 'General medical practice as a career among 1977 Scottish graduates', *Health Bulletin* 44 (6): 351-6.

*— (1989) 'Careers of doctors qualifying in the United Kingdom in 1977: a report on their employment status in 1982' (unpublished).

*Ellin, D.J., Parkhouse, H.F. and Parkhouse, J. (1986) 'Career preferences of doctors qualifying in the United Kingdom in 1983', *Health Trends* 18 (3):

59-63.

Epstein, C.F. and Coeser, R.L. (eds) (1982) *Access to Power: Cross National Studies of Women and Elites*, London: Allen & Unwin.

Evered, D.C., Anderson, J., Griggs, P. and Wakeford, R. (1987) 'The correlates of research success', *British Medical Journal* 295: 241-6.

*Faragher, E.B., Parkhouse, J. and Parkhouse, H.F. (1980) 'Career preferences of doctors qualifying in the United Kingdom in 1978', *Health Trends* 12 (4): 34-5.

Flynn, C.A. and Gardner, F. (1969) 'The careers of women graduates from the Royal Free Hospital Medical School', *British Journal of Medical Education* 3: 28-42.

Fogarty, M., Allen, I. and Walters, P. (1981) *Women in Top Jobs 1968-1979*, Policy Studies Institute, London: Heinemann Education.

Forsyth, G. (1966) *Doctors and State Medicine: A Study of the British Health Service*, 2nd edn 1973, London: Pitman Medical (Open University Set Book).

Furnham, A.F. (1986) 'Medical students' beliefs about nine different specialties', *British Medical Journal* 293: 1,607-10.

Galbraith, J.K. (1989) 'In pursuit of the simple truth', *Guardian*, Review, 28 July: 3.

Gillie, O. (1988) Report of a meeting in London of women gynaecologists, *Independent*, 15 February: 6.

Gish, O. (1970) 'British doctor migration 1962-67', *British Journal of Medical Education* 4: 279-88.

Glaser, W. (1978) *The Brain Drain: Emigration and Return. Findings of a UNITAR Multinational Comparative Study of Professional Personnel of Developing Countries who Study Abroad*, Oxford: Pergamon Press.

Griffith, E.R. (1983) *NHS Management Inquiry Report*, London: DHSS.

Hall, T.L. (1978) 'Supply', in T.L. Hall and A. Mejia (eds) *Health Manpower Planning: Principles, Methods, Issues*, Geneva: World Health Organization.

Harman, H. (1989) Parliamentary Report, *Guardian*, 3 July.

Harris, P.F. (1986) 'Intercalated degrees', *British Medical Journal* 293: 202.

Hutt, R. (1976) 'Doctors' career choice: previous research and its relevance for policy-making', *Medical Education* 10: 463-73.

Hutt, R., Parsons, D. and Pearson, R. (1979) *The Determinants of Doctors' Career Decisions*, a report by the Institute of Manpower Studies to the Department of Health and Social Security and the Scottish Home and Health Department, Brighton: Institute of Manpower Studies, University of Sussex.

Johnson, M.L. and Elston, M.A. (1978) 'Medical Careers', unpublished SSRC Report.

Last, J.M. and Broadie, E. (1970) 'Further careers of young British doctors', *British Medical Journal* i: 735-8.

Last, J.M. and Stanley, G.R. (1968) 'Career preferences of young British doctors', *British Journal of Medical Education* 2: 137-55.

Lawrie, J.E., Newhouse, M.L. and Elliott, P.M. (1966) 'Working capacity of women doctors', *British Medical Journal* i: 409-12.

Lefford, F. (1987) 'Women in medicine – Women doctors: a quarter-century track record', *Lancet* 1: 1,254-6.

Longmore, H.J.A. (1986) 'Intercalated degrees', *British Medical Journal* 293: 202.

Lorber, J. (1984) *Women Physicians: Career Status and Power*, London: Tavistock.

MacFarlene, R.G. and Parry, K.M. (1979) 'Survey of the career experience and postgraduate training of the 1965 and 1970 graduates of the Scottish university medical schools', *Medical Education* 13: 34-8.

MacGowan, A.P., Johnston, P.W. and Thomson, A.W. (1986) 'Intercalated degrees', *British Medical Journal* 293: 201-2.

*McLaughlin, C. and Parkhouse, J. (1972) 'Career preferences of 1971 graduates of two British medical schools', *Lancet* ii: 1,018-20.

*— (1974) 'Career preferences', *Lancet* i: 870-1.

Martin, F.M. and Boddy, F.A. (1962) 'Patterns of career choice and professional attitudes among medical students', in P. Halnos (ed.) *Sociology and Medicine*, Keele: University of Keele (Sociological Review Monograph no. 5).

Milne, T. (1984) 'Personal View', *British Medical Journal* ii: 623.

Nicholl, J.P., Beeby, N.R. and Williams, B.T. (1989) 'Role of the private sector in elective surgery in England and Wales, 1986', *British Medical Journal* 298: 243-7.

Nicol, E.F. (1987) 'Job sharing in general practice', *British Medical Journal* 295: 888-90.

Oakley, C. (1976) 'Pressure of work on doctors and family', *British Medical Journal* ii: 541-2.

*Parkhouse, H.F. and Parkhouse, J. (1989a) 'Women, life and medicine: Achieving a balance – An account of 1974 women medical graduates in 1987', *Community Medicine* 11: 320-35.

*Parkhouse, H.F. and Parkhouse, J. (1990) 'Emigration patterns among 1974 British medical graduates', *Medical Education* 24: 382-8.

Parkhouse, J. (1965) *A New Look at Anaesthetics*, London: Pitman Medical.

*— (1976a) 'Where do graduates do their house jobs?', *Medical Education* 10: 408-9.

*— (1976b) 'A follow-up of career preferences', *Medical Education* 10: 480-2.

— (1978) *Medical Manpower in Britain*, Edinburgh: Churchill Livingstone.

*— (1980) 'Studies of career choice, and career progress', *Health Trends* 12 (2): 34-5.

— (1988) 'On the state of our postgraduate examinations', *Hospital Update* 14 (2): 1,226-9.

*— (1989a) 'Career paths in general practice', *Update* 15 April: 924-7.

— (1989b) 'Manpower planning and training in internal medicine and allied

specialties: a UK case study', *Quarterly Journal, Centre de Sociologie et de Démographie Medicales*, Paris, XXIX année, 2: 137-75.
*Parkhouse, J. and Campbell, M.G. (1983) 'Popularity of geriatrics among Newcastle qualifiers at pre-registration stage', *Lancet* ii: 221.
*— (1984) 'What do young doctors think of their training and themselves?', *British Medical Journal* 288: 1,976-7.
Parkhouse, J. and Darton, R.A. (1979) 'Specialist medical training in Britain: a survey of the hospital specialties in 1975', University of Manchester, Health Services Management Unit, Department of Administration, Working Paper no. 16.
*Parkhouse, J. and Ellin, D.J. (1988a) 'Reasons for doctors' career choice and change of choice', *British Medical Journal* 296: 1,651-3.
— (1988b) 'Intercalated degrees', unpublished observations.
*— (1989) 'Postgraduate qualifications of British doctors', *Medical Education* 23 (3): 348-63.
*— (1990a) 'Internal migration of British doctors: Who goes where?', *Journal of Public Health Medicine* 12: 66-72.
*— (1990b) 'Anaesthetics: career choices and experiences', *Medical Education* 24: 52-67.
*— (1990c) 'Medicine as a career among 1974 and 1977 British medical qualifiers', *Journal of the Royal College of Physicians of London* 24: 178-83.
— (1990d) 'Surgery: career choices and experiences', (unpublished).
— (1990e) 'Psychiatry: career choices and experiences', (unpublished).
*Parkhouse, J. and Howard, M. (1978) 'A follow-up of the career preferences of Manchester and Sheffield graduates of 1972 and 1973', *Medical Education* 12: 377-81.
*Parkhouse, J. and McLaughlin, C. (1975a) 'Career preferences of 1973 graduates', *Lancet* i: 1,342.
— (1975b) *Feasibility Study on Postgraduate Medical Education*, Proceedings Series no. 10, Southend-on-Sea: Institute of Mathematics and its Applications.
*— (1976) 'Career preferences of doctors graduating in 1974', *British Medical Journal* ii: 630-2.
*Parkhouse, J. and Palmer, M.K. (1977) 'Career preferences of doctors qualifying in 1975', *British Medical Journal* ii: 25-7.
*— (1979) 'Career preferences of doctors qualifying in Britain in 1976', *Health Trends* 11 (1): 4-6.
*Parkhouse, J. and Parkhouse, H.F. (1989b) 'Doctors qualifying from United Kingdom medical schools during the calendar years 1977 and 1983', *Medical Education* 23 (1): 62-9.
*Parkhouse, J., Palmer, M.K. and Hambleton, B.A. (1979) 'Career preferences of doctors qualifying in the United Kingdom in 1977', *Health Trends* 11 (2): 35-7.
*Parkhouse, J., Parkhouse, H.F., Hambleton, B.A. and Bullock, N. (1981a)

'Careers of doctors qualifying in Britain in 1974: a follow-up in 1979', *Health Trends* 13 (2): 51-6.

*Parkhouse, J., Campbell, M.G., Parkhouse, H.F. and Philips, P.R. (1981b) 'Career preferences of doctors qualifying in the United Kingdom in 1979', *Health Trends* 13 (4): 103-5.

*Parkhouse, J., Campbell, M.G. and Parkhouse, H.F. (1982) 'Careers of doctors qualifying in Britain in 1974: a report on their employment status in 1979', *British Medical Journal* 285: 522-6.

*— (1983a) 'Career preferences of doctors qualifying in 1974-80: a comparison of pre-registration findings', *Health Trends* 15 (2): 29-35.

*Parkhouse, J., Campbell, M.G., Hambleton, B.A. and Philips, P.R. (1983b) 'Career preferences of doctors qualifying in the United Kingdom in 1980', *Health Trends* 15 (1): 12-14.

Parkhouse, J., Bennett, D. and Ross, J. (1987) 'Medical staffing and training in the West Midlands region', *British Medical Journal* 294: 914-16.

*Parkhouse, J., Ellin, D.J. and Parkhouse, H.F. (1988) 'The views of doctors on management and administration', *Community Medicine* 10 (1): 19-32.

Powell, J. Enoch (1966) *Medicine and Politics 1975 and After*, London: Pitman Medical.

Report (1969) 'Hospital staffing structure (medical and dental): Progress Report on discussions between representatives of the Health Departments and the Joint Consultants Committee', *British Medical Journal Supplement* 4: 53-4.

*Rhodes, P.J. (1989a) 'The career aspirations of women doctors who qualified in 1974 and 1977 from a United Kingdom medical school', *Medical Education* 23 (2): 125-35.

— (1989b) '"Unemployment": what's in a word? Unemployment among doctors who qualified from a United Kingdom medical school in 1974' (unpublished).

*— (1989c) 'What do doctors think of their training? The "Medical" model' (unpublished).

*— (1990) 'Medical women in the middle: family or career? Periods not working and part-time work amongst women doctors who qualified in 1974 and 1977', *Health Trends* 22 (No. 1): 31-4.

Robbins Report (1963) *Report of the Committee on Higher Education*, Cmnd 2154, London: HMSO.

Royal Commission on Medical Education 1965-8 (1968) Report (Todd Report), Cmnd 3569, London: HMSO.

Schumacher, C.F. (1964) 'Personal characteristics of students choosing different types of medical careers', *Journal of Medical Education* 39: 278-8.

Scottish Council for Postgraduate Medical Education (1978) *Career Experience and Postgraduate Training – Report of a Survey of the 1965 and 1970 Graduates of the Scottish University Medical Schools*, Edinburgh: SCPME.

Seale, J. (1966) 'Medical emigration from Great Britain and Ireland since 1962', *British Medical Journal* ii: 576-8.

Secretaries of State for Health (Wales, Northern Ireland and Scotland) (1989)

Working for Patients, Cmnd 555, London: HMSO.

Shapiro, M.C., Western, J.S. and Anderson, D.S. (1988) 'Career preferences and career outcomes of Australian medical students', *Medical Education* 22: 214-21.

Singleton, D. (1988) 'Tomorrows', *Guardian*, 18 May.

Smith, D.J. (1980) *Overseas Doctors in the National Health Service*, London: Policy Studies Institute.

Smith, R. (1986) 'A senseless sacrifice: the fate of intercalated degrees', *British Medical Journal* 292: 1,619-20.

— (1988) 'Medical researchers: training and straining', *British Medical Journal* 296: 920-4.

Social Services Committee (1981) *Medical Education*, Fourth report from the House of Commons Social Services Committee, London: HMSO.

— (1985) *Medical Education Report: Follow-up*, Fifth report from the House of Commons Social Services Committee, London: HMSO.

Spencer, A. and Podmore, D. (eds) (1987) *In a Man's World: Essays on Women in Male Dominated Professions*, London: Tavistock.

Wakeford, R., Lyon, J., Evered, D. and Sanders, N. (1985) 'Where do medically qualified researchers come from?', *Lancet* ii: 262-5.

Walton, H. (ed.) (1986) 'Education and training in psychiatry: a case study in the continuity of medical education', King Edward's Hospital Fund for London.

Ward, A., Francis, B., Dawson, C., Ennis, E. and Morrison, J. (1981) *Careers for Medical Women*, Sheffield: University of Sheffield Medical School.

Ward, A.W.M. (1982) 'Careers of medical women', *British Medical Journal* 284: 31-3.

— (1984) 'Psychiatrists who passed the MRC Psych 1975-77', *Health Trends* 16: 80-3.

Wattis, J., Wattis, L. and Arie, T. (1981) 'Psychogeriatrics: a national survey of a new branch of psychiatry', *British Medical Journal* 282: 1,529-33.

Willink Report (1957) *Report of the Committee to consider the Future Numbers of Medical Practitioners and the Appropriate Intake of Medical Students*, London: HMSO.

Wills, L.A.M. (1986) 'Women in medicine', *British Medical Journal* 293: 567.

World Health Organization (1985) *Medical Specialization in Relation to Health Needs*, report on a WHO meeting, Abano Terme, Italy, 22-25 October 1984, Copenhagen: WHO.

Wyllie, A.H. and Currie, A.R. (1986) 'The Edinburgh intercalated honours BSc in pathology: evaluation of selection methods, undergraduate performance, and postgraduate career', *British Medical Journal* 292: 1,646-8.

Index

Note: Page references in italics indicate tables and figures.